Clinical Trials in Age-Related Macular Degeneration Treatment

Jeffrey N. Weiss

Clinical Trials in Age-Related Macular Degeneration Treatment

Springer

Jeffrey N. Weiss
Parkland, FL, USA

ISBN 978-3-031-58802-0 ISBN 978-3-031-58803-7 (eBook)
https://doi.org/10.1007/978-3-031-58803-7

This Springer imprint is published by the registered company Springer Nature Switzerland AG
The registered company address is: Gewerbestrasse 11, 6330 Cham, Switzerland

For the patients that have allowed us the privilege to serve.

Preface

This book is a compendium of the worldwide ocular stem cell, gene therapy, pharmaceutical, and other miscellaneous studies treating Age-Related Macular Degeneration registered with Clinicaltrials.gov. Clinicaltrials.gov is the largest website listing of registered clinical research studies in the world. The information presented is accurate as of November 2023. I have divided the studies into multiple categories: Completed, Active/Recruiting, Active/Not-Recruiting, Not Yet Recruiting, and Enrolling by Invitation. Regarding study location, United States locations are listed first, followed by other countries in alphabetical order. As studies have many sites, frequently in many countries, the sponsor location is used.

I corrected the mischaracterization of studies, only included those that truly belonged within each category, removed extraneous information, and corrected spelling and grammar, in order to produce a consistent and easy-to-read format. The Study and the Clinical Trial number are provided to make it easier for the reader to obtain further information.

I hope that by providing this reference, the field of age-related macular degeneration treatment will be advanced.

Parkland, FL, USA Jeffrey N. Weiss

Contents

Chapter 1
Introduction to Age-Related Macular Degeneration

Age-related macular degeneration (AMD) is the leading cause of visual loss in the elderly population. The hallmark of AMD is the presence of drusen, which are composed of lipids, proteins, lipofuscin granules, and small RNAs. The late stage of AMD may be divided into a "wet" or neovascular type, and the much more common "dry" or atrophic type also called geographic atrophy. Currently, there are effective treatments in the form of Vascular Endothelial Growth Factor Inhibitors, laser photocoagulation, and photodynamic therapy for patients with wet AMD, but there is no effective treatment for the dry type of AMD.

Smoking, obesity, and high-fat diets have been shown to impact the development and progression of AMD. Initially, dietary supplements, such as lutein, zeaxanthin, and omega-3 fatty acids, were shown to slow AMD progression but further analysis did not prove efficacy.

Visual cycle modulators, inflammatory modulators, and neuroprotective agents have all been studied in an attempt to slow the progression of dry AMD. Oxidative and mitochondrial stresses are postulated to promote the development and progression of AMD but no effective pharmacological interventions have proven successful.

Fifty percent of the risk of developing AMD has been explained by a complex association of genetics, environment, and lifestyle. Genetic linkage analysis has identified multiple sets of genetic variants that have roles in immune response, inflammatory processes, and retinal homeostasis.

Replacement of the retinal pigment epithelium (RPE) using cell-based therapies has been performed but this technique relies upon the presence of remaining photoreceptors. Treating significant geographic atrophy, with the loss of all the retinal layers, remains problematic. Difficulties include the formation of functional synapses, and the successful orientation and polarization of the donor photoreceptors following transplantation.

In this book, we explore the various potential therapies being evaluated in the treatment of both neovascular AMD and geographic atrophy.

J. N. Weiss, *Clinical Trials in Age-Related Macular Degeneration Treatment*,
https://doi.org/10.1007/978-3-031-58803-7_1

Further Reading

Harris JR, Fisher R, Jorgensen M, et al. CD 133 progenitor cells from the bone marrow contribute to retinal pigment epithelial repair. Stem Cells. 2009;27(2):457–66.

Gong L, Wu Q, Song B, Lu B, Zhang Y. Differentiation of rat mesenchymal stem cells transplanted into the subretinal space of sodium iodate-injected rats. Clin Experiment Ophthalmol. 2008;36:666–71.

Jiang Y, Zhang Y, Zhang L, et al. Therapeutic effect of bone marrow mesenchymal stem cells on laser-induced retinal injury in mice. Int J Mol Sci. 2014;15:9372–85.

Becker S, Jayaram H, Limb GA. Recent advances towards the clinical application of stem cells for retinal regeneration. Cells. 2012;1:851–73.

Pesaresi M, Bonila-Pons SA, Simonte G, et al. Endogenous mobilization of bone-marrow cells into the murine retina induces fusion-mediated reprograming of Müller glia cells. EBioMedicine. 2018;30:38–51.

Schmier JK, Covert DW, Lau EC. Patterns and costs associated with progression of age-related macular degeneration. Am J Ophthalmol. 2012;154(4):675–81.

Wong WT, Chakravarthy U, Klein R, Mitchell P, et al. The natural history and prognosis of neovascular age-related macular degeneration: a systematic review of the literature and meta-analysis. Ophthalmology. 2008;115(1):116–26.

Buschini E, Fea AM, Lavia C, Nassisi M, et al. Recent developments in the management of dry age-related macular degeneration. Clin Ophthalmol. 2015;9:563–74.

Cheung LK, Eaton A. Age-related macular degeneration. Pharmacotherapy. 2013;33(8):838–55.

Chew EY, Clemons TE, Agron E, Sperduto RD, et al. Age-relate eye disease study research: ten-year follow-up of age-related macular degeneration in the age-related eye disease study: AREDS report no. 36. JAMA Ophthalmol. 2014;132(3):272–7.

Suter M, Reme C, Grimm C, Wenzel A, et al. Age-related macular degeneration. The lipofusion component N-retinyl-N-retinylidene ethanolamine detaches proapoptotic proteins from mitochondria and induces apoptosis ibn mammalian retinal pigment epithelial cells. J Biol Chem. 2000;275(50):39625–30.

Baudouin C, Peyman GA, Fredj-Reygrobellet D, Gordon WC, et al. Immunohistological study of subretinal membranes in age-related macular degeneration. Jpn J Ophthalmol. 1992;36(4):443–51.

Danis RP, Lavine JA, Domalpally A. Geographic atrophy in patients with advanced dry age-related macular degeneration: current challenges and future prospects. Clin Ophthalmol. 2015;9:2159–74.

Maller J, et al. Common variation in three genes, including a noncoding variant in CFH, strongly influences risk of age-related macular degeneration. Nat Genet. 2006;38:1055–9.

Schwartz SD, Regillo CD, Lam BL, Eliott D, et al. Human embryonic stem cell-derived retinal pigment epithelium in patients with age-related macular degeneration and Stargardt's macular dystrophy: follow-up of two open-label phase ½ studies. Lancet. 2015;385(9967):509–16.

Forest DL, Johnson LV, Clegg DO. Cellular models and therapies for age-related macular degeneration. Dis Model Mech. 2015;8(5):421–7.

Song WJ, Park KM, Kim HJ, et al. Treatment of macular degeneration using embryonic stem cell-derived retinal pigment epithelium: preliminary results in Asian patients. Stem Cell Rep. 2015;4(5):860–72.

Weiss JN, Levy S. Stem cell ophthalmology treatment study (SCOTS): bone marrow derived stem cells in the treatment of age-related macular degeneration. Medicines. 2020;7:16. https://doi.org/10.3390/medicines7040016, 1–13.

Chapter 2
Tables

See Tables 2.1, 2.2 and 2.3.

At present there are 9 Stem Cell studies, 14 Gene Therapy studies, and 25 “Other” studies recruiting for AMD trials listed on clinicaltrials.gov. Of the 48 worldwide studies, 6 Stem Cell studies utilize a proprietary product (67%), 13 Gene Therapy studies utilize a proprietary product (93%), and 22 “Other” studies utilize a proprietary product (88%).

One study was U.S. National Eye Institute (NEI) supported (2%), 2 studies were patient funded (4%), and 12 studies were University/Hospital supported (25%). Sixty-nine percent of studies were corporate funded.

It is curious that in the United States, where millions of dollars in grants and donations are made for research, there was only 1 NEI-supported study, and no university/hospital-funded studies. Is the money being spent on research for other conditions, or is the work not being employed in a practical manner resulting in a clinical study?

J. N. Weiss, *Clinical Trials in Age-Related Macular Degeneration Treatment*,
https://doi.org/10.1007/978-3-031-58803-7_2

Table 2.1 Stem cell studies

	United States	Caribbean	China	Great Britain
Number of Studies	4	1	2	2
Non-Proprietary	1		2	
Proprietary	3	1		2
Support				
Corporate	2			
University/Hospital			2	2
NEI	1			
No Support	1	1		
Phase Not Applicable	1		1	1
Phase 1	1	1	1	1
Phase 1/2	2			
Phase 2				
Phase 2/3				
Phase 3				

Table 2.2 Gene studies

	United States	Canada	China
Number of Studies	7	1	6
Non-Proprietary			
Proprietary	7	1	5
Support			
Corporate	7		
University/Hospital			1
NEI			
No Support			
Phase Not Applicable			1
Phase 1	1		4
Phase 1/2	2	1	1
Phase 2	2		
Phase 2/3	1		
Phase 3	1		

Table 2.3 "Other treatments" studies

	United States	Australia	Austria	China	Italy	Korea	Norway	South America	Thailand
Number of Studies	10	2	2	6	1	1	1	1	1
Drug	8	1	1	6					1
Electrical	1					1			
Laser/Light		1			1		1	1	
Ultrasound	1								
Training			1						
Non-Proprietary	1	1			1				
Proprietary	9	1	2	6		1	1	1	1
Support									
Corporate	9	1		5		1		1	1
University/Hospital	1	1	2	1	1		1		
NEI									
No Support									
Phase Not Applicable	2	1	2		1	1	1	1	
Phase 1	2	1		1					
Phase 1/2									
Phase 2	5			1					1
Phase 2/3									
Phase 3	1			3					
Phase 4			1	1					

Chapter 3
Stem Cell Studies

United States

Recruiting

Safety and Tolerability of RPE Stem Cell-derived RPE (RPESC-RPE) Transplantation in Patients with Dry Age-Related Macular Degeneration (AMD)

ClinicalTrials.gov ID NCT04627428

Sponsor Luxa Biotechnology, LLC
Information provided by Luxa Biotechnology, LLC (Responsible Party)
Last Update Posted 2023-10-05

Study Overview

Brief Summary
The main objective of the study is evaluation of the safety and tolerability of RPESC-RPE-4W as therapy for dry AMD.

Detailed Description
RPESC-RPE-4W is Allogeneic RPE stem cell (RPESC)-derived RPE cells (RPESC-RPE) isolated from the RPE layer of human cadaveric eyes are transplanted under the macular.

This first-in-human Phase 1/2a open-label dose-escalation interventional study plans to enroll a total of 18 subjects.

Official Title
A Phase1/2a, Open-Label Study to Evaluate the Safety and Tolerability of RPE Stem Cell-Derived RPE (RPESC-RPE) Transplantation as Therapy for Dry Age-Related Macular Degeneration (AMD)

J. N. Weiss, *Clinical Trials in Age-Related Macular Degeneration Treatment*,
https://doi.org/10.1007/978-3-031-58803-7_3

Conditions
Dry Age-related Macular Degeneration

Intervention/Treatment
- Biological: RPESC-RPE-4W

Other Study ID Numbers
- RPESC-RPE-01
- U01EY030581 (U.S. NIH Grant/Contract)
- UG3EY031810 (U.S. NIH Grant/Contract)

Study Start (Actual)
2022-04-05

Primary Completion (Estimated)
2025-05-31

Study Completion (Estimated)
2025-05-31

Enrollment (Estimated)
18

Study Type
Interventional

Phase
Phase 1 Phase 2

Study Contact
Name: Jeffrey H Stern, M.D., Ph.D.
Phone Number: 05184371111
Email: jeffreystern@luxabiotech.com

United States
Michigan Locations

Ann Arbor, Michigan, United States, 48105
Recruiting
University of Michigan Kellogg Eye Center

Contact
Rajesh C Rao, M.D.

Eligibility Criteria
Description

Inclusion Criteria
- Clinical diagnosis of dry AMD
- Ability to understand and give informed consent
- Adult male or female >55 years of age

- Medically suitable to undergo vitrectomy and subretinal injection (>60% on Karnofsky scale)
- Postmenopausal if the female (expected to be common for the age limitation), or the female partner of a male subject is unable to father children
- If the male is willing to use barrier and spermicidal contraception during the study

Exclusion Criteria
- Allergy or hypersensitivity to dilation drops or fluorescein
- Active major medical conditions limiting the ability to participate in the study
- Active malignancy or treatment with chemotherapy
- Systemic immunosuppressant therapy within the past six months
- History of toxoplasmosis, retinal histoplasmosis, or tuberculosis
- Receipt of investigational product (IP) in a clinical trial within the prior six months
- Any other medical condition, which, in the Investigator's judgment, will interfere with the subject's ability to comply with the protocol, compromises the subject safety, or interferes with the interpretation of the study results
- Pregnant or nursing females

Ages Eligible for Study
55 Years and older (Adult, Older Adult)

Sexes Eligible for Study
All

Accepts Healthy Volunteers
No

Primary Purpose: Treatment
Allocation: Non-Randomized
Interventional Model: Sequential Assignment
Masking: None (Open Label)

Arms and interventions

Participant group/arm	Intervention/treatment
Experimental: 50,000 cells Six patients will receive a single dose of 50,000 RPESC-RPE-4W cells in the eye	Biological: RPESC-RPE-4W • RPESC-RPE-4W
Experimental: 150,000 cells Six patients will receive a single dose of 150,000 RPESC-RPE-4W cells in the eye	Biological: RPESC-RPE-4W • RPESC-RPE-4W
Experimental: 250,000 cells Six patients will receive a single dose of 250,000 RPESC-RPE-4W cells in the eye	Biological: RPESC-RPE-4W • RPESC-RPE-4W

Primary outcome measures

Outcome measure	Measure description	Time frame
Safety and tolerability of RPESC-RPE-4W transplantation	The transplantation of RPESC-RPE-4W cells will be considered safe and tolerated in the absence of: • Decrease in visual acuity (VA) of more than 15 Early Treatment Diabetic Retinopathy Study (ETDRS) letters (or to worse than counting fingers at three feet) from baseline • Any Grade 2 (CTCAE version 5) or greater adverse events (AE) related to the cell product and investigational interventions. • Any evidence that the cells are contaminated with an infectious agent or serious immune response to the cell product • Any evidence that the cells show tumorigenic potential	24 months

Secondary outcome measures

Outcome measure	Measure description	Time frame
Change in the mean of best-corrected visual acuity (BCVA)	Change in visual acuity will be measured by the ETDRS chart	24 months
Loss of ≥10 decibels of ten-degree average visual sensitivity microperimetry	Loss of ≥10 decibels of ten-degree average visual sensitivity will be measured by microperimetry	24 months
Change in GA lesion area	Change in GA lesion area will be measured	24 months
Evidence of structural changes	Structural evidence will be measured by OCT imaging, autofluorescence, fluorescein angiography, and fundus photography	24 months

Sponsor

Luxa Biotechnology, LLC

Collaborators

- National Institutes of Health (NIH)
- National Eye Institute (NEI)
- Regenerative Research Foundation

Investigators

- Principal Investigator: Rajesh C Rao, M.D., University of Michigan Kellogg Eye Center

General Publications

No publications available

United States

Recruiting

Autologous Transplantation of Induced Pluripotent Stem Cell-Derived Retinal Pigment Epithelium for Geographic Atrophy Associated with Age-Related Macular Degeneration

ClinicalTrials.gov ID NCT04339764

Sponsor National Eye Institute (NEI)
Information provided by the National Institutes of Health Clinical Center (CC) (National Eye Institute (NEI)) (Responsible Party)
Last Update Posted 2023-05-12

Study Overview

Brief Summary
Background
Age-related macular degeneration is a common eye disease in people over 50. The "dry" form of the disease can worsen into geographic atrophy, causing blind spots. Researchers want to learn if replacing older eye cells with younger ones can help treat this disease.

Objective
To test the safety of putting cells inside the eye as a possible future treatment for dry age-related macular degeneration.

Eligibility
People ages 55 and older who have geographic atrophy with loss of vision. People who have had "wet" macular degeneration in either eye are NOT eligible.

Design
Participants will be screened with:

- Medical history
- Physical exam
- Blood and urine tests
- Eye exam
- Eye photos
- Fluorescein angiography. An intravenous (IV) line is placed in an arm vein. A dye is injected. A camera takes pictures of the dye as it flows through the eyes' blood vessels.
- Electroretinography. An electrode is taped to the participant's forehead. They sit in the dark. After 30 min, numbing eye drops and contact lenses are placed in their eyes. They watch flashing lights.
- Tuberculosis test

- Chest X-ray
- Electrocardiography. Sticky pads are placed on participants' chests to record the heart's electrical activity.

Participants will have at least 14 study visits over 5 and a half years. They will repeat screening tests.

Participants will have retinal pigment epithelium (RPE) transplantation surgery in one eye. For this, cells from participants' blood are turned into RPE cells. These cells are placed in their eye through a cut in their retina. They will get dilating eye drops, an IV line, and anesthesia that may make them sleep. A gas bubble will be put in their eye to help it heal.

Participants will be contacted yearly for up to 15 years.

Detailed Description

Age-related macular degeneration (AMD) is a leading cause of vision loss among the elderly. There is no treatment for geographic atrophy (GA), the advanced stage of dry AMD, in which cells of the neurosensory retina and associated retinal pigment epithelium (RPE) gradually degenerate and die. Advances in stem cell biology allowing differentiation of pluripotent cells into RPE in vitro make feasible a cell-based strategy for the potential treatment of AMD, and recent methods for induced pluripotent stem cell (iPSC) the generation offer the promise of individualized autologous therapy. Such an approach involves the generation of iPSC from somatic cells taken from a patient with GA, differentiation of iPSC into RPE grown as a monolayer on a thin scaffold in vitro, and transplantation of the RPE/scaffold construct into a small region in the subretinal space of the same patient, with a goal of rescuing the overlying neurosensory retina from further degeneration.

Objective

To evaluate the safety and feasibility of subretinal transplantation of iPSC-derived RPE, grown as a monolayer on a biodegradable poly lactic-co-glycolic acid (PLGA) scaffold, as a potential autologous cell-based therapy for GA associated with AMD.

Study Population: Five participants will undergo RPE transplantation in one eye. Eligible eyes will have GA, best-corrected visual acuity (BCVA) between 20/100 and inclusive of counting fingers (CF), and a fellow eye that has the same or better BCVA. If the National Eye Institute (NEI) Data and Safety Monitoring Committee (DSMC) gives clearance to proceed based on a review of data from the first cohort, a second cohort of up to seven additional participants with GA, BCVA between 20/80 and CF (inclusive) in the eye being considered for RPE transplantation, and same or better visual acuity in the other eye may undergo the procedure to gather additional safety and potential efficacy data useful for planning future studies. Up to 20 participants may be enrolled to allow for screening failures, for participants withdrawing from the study prior to RPE transplantation, or cases where the RPE cell transplantation does not occur due to intraoperative surgical considerations.

Design

In this Phase I/IIa, prospective, single-arm, single-center clinical trial, participants will undergo subretinal transplantation of autologous iPSC-derived RPE in one eye and will be followed for five years after surgery.

Outcome Measures

The primary outcome measure is the safety of RPE/PLGA transplantation, as determined by the assessment of visual acuity change and summary of adverse events at 12 months after RPE/PLGA transplantation. Secondary outcome measures include visual acuity change and adverse event reporting at 24 and 60 months, and changes in the following at 12, 24, and 60 months as compared with baseline, assessed in the transplanted region, and compared where applicable with other areas in the macula, and/or with corresponding regions in the fellow eye: retinal sensitivity and fixation parameters assessed by microperimetry; multifocal electroretinography (mfERG) responses; macular structure on cross-sectional and en face imaging by optical coherence tomography (OCT); macular features on color, single-wavelength reflectance, and fundus autofluorescence (FAF) photography; and fluorescein angiography (FA). Some NEI participants may undergo imaging of photoreceptor/RPE features using adaptive-optics-assisted macular imaging under a separate protocol (e.g., 15-EI-0020).

Official Title

A Phase I/IIa Trial for Autologous Transplantation of Induced Pluripotent Stem Cell-Derived Retinal Pigment Epithelium for Geographic Atrophy Associated With Age-Related Macular Degeneration

Conditions

Age-Related Macular Degeneration

Intervention/Treatment

- Drug: iPSC-derived RPE/PLGA transplantation

Other Study ID Numbers

- 200052
- 20-EI-0052

Study Start (Actual)

2020-09-23

Primary Completion (Estimated)

2029-05-31

Study Completion (Estimated)

2029-05-31

Enrollment (Estimated)

20

Study Type

Interventional

Phase
Phase 1 Phase 2

Study Contact
Name: Angel H Garced, R.N.
Phone Number: (301) 594-3141
Email: angel.garced@nih.gov

Study Contact Backup
Name: M. Teresa Magone de Quadros Costa, M.D.
Phone Number: (301) 435-4562
Email: teresa.magonedequadroscosta@nih.gov
United States
Maryland Locations

Bethesda, Maryland, United States, 20892
Recruiting
National Institutes of Health Clinical Center

Contact
For more information at the NIH Clinical Center contact the Office of Patient Recruitment (OPR)
800-411-1222 ext TTY8664111010 prpl@cc.nih.gov

Eligibility Criteria
Description

Inclusion Criteria
To be eligible, the following inclusion criteria must be met, where applicable.

- Participants must be 55 years of age or older
- Participants must have a diagnosis of AMD, defined as the presence (or history, as documented in available color fundus photographs) of at least one medium or large druse (greater than or equal to 63-micrometer diameter) in the macula in at least one eye; and the presence of GA in at least one eye.
- Participants must understand and sign the protocol informed consent document.
- Any participant of childbearing potential must have a negative pregnancy test at screening and must be willing to undergo pregnancy testing prior to RPE transplantation.
- Any participant of childbearing potential and any participant able to father children must have (or have a partner who has) had a hysterectomy or vasectomy, be completely abstinent from intercourse, or must agree to practice an effective method of contraception through Month 12 in the study. Acceptable methods of contraception include:
  - Hormonal contraception (i.e., birth control pills, injected hormones, dermal patch, or vaginal ring)
  - Intrauterine device
  - Barrier methods (diaphragm, condom) with spermicide or
  - Surgical sterilization (tubal ligation)

- Participants must be medically able to comply with the study treatment (including the ability to safely receive anesthesia for surgery), study testing and procedures, and follow-up visits.

Study Eye Inclusion Criteria

- The study eye must have one or more regions of geographic atrophy with a total area of 1 disc area or more. A region of geographic atrophy is defined as an area of uniform hypofluorescence on fundus autofluorescence (FAF) imaging, with greatest linear dimension at least 500 micrometers, with a border within 500 micrometers of the foveal center, not compatible with pigmentary changes, drusen, RPE detachment, drusenoid RPE detachment, hemorrhage, or another lesion. (Note: If macular geographic atrophy is contiguous with peripapillary atrophy, complicating the calculation of total area, only atrophy temporal to a vertical line placed a half-disc diameter temporal to the temporal border of the disc will be included in the total area of geographic atrophy calculated for eligibility purposes.)
- For participants in the first cohort, the study eye must have an ETDRS best-corrected visual acuity (BCVA) letter score of less than or equal to 53 and greater than or equal to CF (i.e., Snellen equivalent between 20/100 and CF), and the fellow eye must have a letter score no more than five letters worse than the study eye using Electronic Visual Acuity (EVA) testing. (Note: Letter scores within five or fewer letters of each other are accordingly considered equal for eligibility determination, and other factors may be used to select the study eye if both are eligible by BCVA.)
- For participants in the second cohort, the study eye must have an ETDRS best-corrected visual acuity (BCVA) letter score of less than or equal to 58 and greater than or equal to CF (i.e., Snellen equivalent between 20/80 and CF), and the fellow eye must have a letter score no more than five letters worse than the study eye using Electronic Visual Acuity (EVA) testing. (Note: Letter scores within five or fewer letters of each other are accordingly considered equal for eligibility determination, and other factors may be used to select the study eye if both are eligible by BCVA.)
- The compromise in visual acuity for the study eye must be judged predominantly secondary to dry AMD, in the judgment of the investigator.
- The study eye must have clarity of ocular media and a degree of pupil dilation sufficient to permit adequate fundus photography and safe vitrectomy surgery.
- The study eye must be either pseudophakic or aphakic.

Exclusion Criteria

A participant is not eligible if any of the following exclusion criteria are present:

- Participant is actively receiving another study medication/investigational product (IP).
- Participant has any condition that significantly increases the risk of systemic corticosteroids or systemic steroid-sparing immuno-modulatory agents, such as uncontrolled diabetes mellitus, chronic hepatitis or liver failure, chronic renal failure, or present infection with HIV, syphilis, tuberculosis, hepatitis B, or hepa-

titis C (past infection now resolved, where applicable, is not exclusionary; but persistent infection, even if latent, is exclusionary).

- Participant has a diagnosis of a malignancy expected to affect two-year survival.
- Participant is pregnant, breastfeeding, or planning to become pregnant through the first 12 months of the study.
- Participant has a family history of a retinal degeneration other than AMD suspected to play a role in the ocular phenotype of the participant in the judgment of the investigator, based on disease features and mode of inheritance, such as in a case of autosomal dominant retinal degeneration in a parent or child.
- Participant is taking, or has taken within the previous year, medication with known potential toxicity to the retina, optic nerve, or lens (such as chloroquine, hydroxychloroquine, and ethambutol).
- Participant is unable or unwilling to give informed consent that includes the use of medical records and clinical samples for current and future research.

Study/Eye Exclusion Criteria

- The study eye must not have macular subretinal or choroidal neovascularization, as assessed by FA and OCT; or any history of such neovascularization (as assessed by past available records or images).
- The study eye must not have any serous or hemorrhagic pigment epithelial detachment, as assessed by FA and OCT.
- The study eye must not have any history of photodynamic therapy (PDT) or macular thermal laser photocoagulation, or history of intravitreal injection of anti-vascular endothelial growth factor (VEGF) agents or corticosteroids (excepting medications used peri-operatively at prior cataract surgery).
- The study eye must not have an axial length > 25.0 mm.
- The study eye must not have had any surgery in the previous 12 weeks, or laser capsulotomy in the previous four weeks.
- The study eye must not have chronic glaucoma; or significant ocular hypertension, defined as documented intraocular pressure of greater than or equal to 26 mmHg on at least two occasions in the absence of self-limited acute glaucoma; or a history of probable or definite steroid response manifesting as acute glaucoma or ocular hypertension, even if self-limited and no longer present; and the fellow eye must not have evidence for present or past glaucoma or ocular hypertension judged to significantly impact the risk of glaucoma in the study eye (including history of probable or definite steroid response). (Note: History of self-limited acute glaucoma in a study or fellow eye, if not secondary to steroid response, and if now resolved and not expected to recur (e.g., history of elevated intraocular pressure from retained visco-elastic after cataract surgery), is not exclusionary. History of glaucoma or ocular hypertension in the fellow eye, if not felt to significantly impact the risk of glaucoma in the study eye, is not exclusionary.)
- The study eye must not have a condition materially increasing the risks of surgery or potentially affecting visual function over the next two years in the judgment of the investigator, such as chronic uveitis, diabetic retinopathy, ker-

atitis, scleritis, optic neuropathy, untreated retinal detachment, macular edema from prior vein occlusion or other cause, proliferative vitreoretinopathy (PVR), vitreous hemorrhage, and pathologic myopia. A history of such conditions is not exclusionary, if judged to not materially increase risks of surgery or to potentially affect vision in the next two years in the opinion of the investigator.

Ages Eligible for Study
55 Years and older (Adult, Older Adult)

Sexes Eligible for Study
All

Accepts Healthy Volunteers
No
Study Plan

Design Details
Primary Purpose: Treatment
Allocation: N/A
Interventional Model: Single Group Assignment
Masking: None (Open Label)

Arms and interventions

Participant group/arm	Intervention/treatment
Experimental: Participants receiving intervention Participants receiving intervention	Drug: iPSC-derived RPE/PLGA transplantation • iPSC-derived RPE/PLGA transplantation

Primary outcome measures

Outcome measure	Measure description	Time frame
Visual acuity change	Safety measure	12, 24, and 60 month
Summary of adverse events	Safety measure	12, 24, and 60 month

Secondary outcome measures

Outcome measure	Measure description	Time frame
Retinal Structure (optical coherence tomography)	Safety and efficacy measure	12, 24, and 60 month
Retinal sensitivity and fixation (microperimetry)	Safety and efficacy measure	12, 24, and 60 month
Multifocal electroretinography responses	Safety and efficacy measure	12, 24, and 60 month
Retinal Structure (color and autofluorescence imaging)	Safety and efficacy measure	12, 24, and 60 month
Retinal structure (fluorescein angiography)	Safety and efficacy measure	12, 24, and 60 month

Sponsor
National Eye Institute (NEI)

Collaborators
No information provided

Investigators
- Principal Investigator: M. Teresa Magone de Quadros Costa, M.D., National Eye Institute (NEI)

General Publications
No publications available

United States

Recruiting

Stem Cell Ophthalmology Treatment Study II (SCOTS2)

ClinicalTrials.gov ID NCT03011541

Sponsor MD Stem Cells
Information provided by MD Stem Cells (Responsible Party)
Last Update Posted 2023-06-06

Study Overview

Brief Summary
This study will evaluate the use of autologous bone marrow derived stem cells (BMSC) for the treatment of retinal and optic nerve damage or disease.

Detailed Description
Eyes with the loss of vision from retinal or optic nerve conditions generally considered irreversible will be treated with a combination of injections of autologous bone marrow derived stem cells isolated from the bone marrow using standard medical and surgical practices. Retinal conditions may include degenerative, ischemic, or physical damage (examples may include macular degeneration, hereditary retinal dystrophies such as retinitis pigmentosa, Stargardt, non-perfusion retinopathies, and post retinal detachment). Optic Nerve conditions may include degenerative, ischemic, or physical damage (examples may include optic nerve damage from glaucoma, compression, ischemic optic neuropathy, optic atrophy). Injections may include retrobulbar, subtenon, intravitreal, intraocular, subretinal, and intravenous. Patients will be followed for 12 months with serial comprehensive eye examinations including relevant imaging and diagnostic ophthalmic testing.

Official Title
Bone Marrow Derived Stem Cell Ophthalmology Treatment Study II

Conditions
Retinal Disease
Age-Related Macular Degeneration
Retinitis Pigmentosa
Stargardt Disease
Optic Neuropathy
Nonarteritic Ischemic Optic Neuropathy
Optic Atrophy
Optic Nerve Disease
Glaucoma
Leber Hereditary Optic Neuropathy
Blindness
Vision Loss Night
Vision Loss Partial
Vision, Low
Retinopathy
Maculopathy
Macular Degeneration
Retina Atrophy

Intervention/Treatment
- Procedure: Arm 1

Other Study ID Numbers
- SCOTS2

Study Start (Actual)
2016-01

Primary Completion (Estimated)
2024-07

Study Completion (Estimated)
2025-07

Enrollment (Estimated)
500

Study Type
Interventional

Phase
Not Applicable

Study Contact
Name: Steven Levy, MD
Phone Number: 203-423-9494
Email: stevenlevy@mdstemcells.com

Study Contact Backup
Name: Steven Levy, MD
Phone Number: 203-423-9494
United States
Connecticut Locations

Westport, Connecticut, United States, 06880
Recruiting
MD Stem Cells

Contact
Steven Levy, MD
203-423-9494 stevenlevy@mdstemcells.com

Contact
Steven Levy, MD
203-423-9494
Sub-Investigator:
Steven Levy, MD

Florida Locations

Coral Springs, Florida, United States, 33065
Recruiting
MD Stem Cells

Contact
Steven Levy, MD
203-423-9494

United Arab Emirates

Dubai, United Arab Emirates
Recruiting
Medcare Orthopaedics & Spine Hospital

Contact
Steven Levy, MD
(001) 2034239494

Eligibility Criteria
Description

Inclusion Criteria
- Have objective, documented damage to the retina or optic nerve unlikely to improve or
- Have objective, documented damage to the retina or optic nerve that is progressive and has less than or equal to 20/30 best-corrected central visual acuity in one or both eyes and/or an abnormal visual field in one or both eyes.
- Be at least 3 months post-surgical treatment intended to treat any ophthalmologic disease and stable.

- If under current medical therapy (pharmacologic treatment) for a retinal or optic nerve disease be considered stable on that treatment and unlikely to have visual function improvement (e.g., glaucoma with intraocular pressure stable on topical medications but visual field damage).
- Have the potential for improvement with BMSC treatment and be at minimal risk of any potential harm from the procedure.
- Be over the age of 18.
- Be medically stable and able to be medically cleared by their primary care physician or a licensed primary care practitioner for the procedure.
- Medical clearance means that in the estimation of the primary care practitioner, the patient can reasonably be expected to undergo the procedure without significant medical risk to health.

Exclusion Criteria

- Patients who are not capable of an adequate ophthalmologic examination or evaluation to document the pathology.
- Patients who are not capable or not willing to undergo follow-up eye exams with the Principal Investigator or their ophthalmologist or optometrist as outlined in the protocol.
- Patients who are not capable of providing informed consent.
- Patients who may be at significant risk to general health or to the eyes and visual function should they undergo the procedure.

Ages Eligible for Study
18 Years and older (Adult, Older Adult)

Sexes Eligible for Study
All

Accepts Healthy Volunteers
No

Design Details
Primary Purpose: Treatment
Allocation: N/A
Interventional Model: Single Group Assignment
Interventional Model Description: Single Arm—Arm 1. Comparator is the natural history of the disease
Masking: None (Open Label)

Arms and interventions

Participant group/arm	Intervention/treatment
Other: Arm 1 BMSC provided retrobulbar, subtenon, and intravenous for one or both eyes	Procedure: Arm 1 • Procedure/Surgery: RB (Retrobulbar) Retrobulbar injection of Bone Marrow Derived Stem Cells (BMSC) Procedure/Surgery: ST (Subtenon) Subtenon injection of Bone Marrow Derived Stem Cells (BMSC) Procedure/Surgery: IV (Intravenous) Intravenous injection of Bone Marrow Derived Stem Cells (BMSC) • Other Names: – Retrobulbar (RB) – Subtenon (ST) – Intravenous (IV)

Primary outcome measures

Outcome measure	Measure description	Time frame
Visual Acuity	Best-corrected visual acuity will be measured with the Snellen Eye Chart and the ETDRS (Early Treatment Diabetic Retinopathy Study) Eye Chart when available at each post-procedure visit. Intervals at a minimum will be a first post-procedure day, then 3, 6, and 12 months post-procedure day. Recommended visit 1 month post-procedure day	Change from pre-procedure to 12 months

Secondary outcome measures

Outcome measure	Measure description	Time frame
Visual Fields	Visual fields will be evaluated with automated perimetry during post-procedure visits as needed and specifically at 6 and 12 months. Visual fields are a key measurement in patients with peripheral vision loss	Change from pre-procedure to 12 months
Optical Coherence Tomography (OCT)	OCT thickness of the retinal nerve fiber layer the optic nerve and/or macula during the post-procedure visits as needed and specifically at 6 and 12 months—if available	Change from pre-procedure to 12 months

Sponsor

MD Stem Cells

Collaborators

No information provided

Investigators

- Study Chair: Steven Levy, MD, MD Stem Cells
- Principal Investigator: Jeffrey Weiss, MD, Coral Springs

General Publications

- Weiss JN, Levy S. The Role of Patient Funded Clinical Research in Advancing Medical Care. ClinicalTrials.gov Identifier: NCT01920867.
- Weiss JN, Levy S, Malkin A. Stem Cell Ophthalmology Treatment Study (SCOTS) for Retinal and Optic Nerve Disease: a Preliminary Report. Neural Regeneration Research. 10;6: 982–988, 2015.
- Weiss JN, Levy S, Benes SC. Stem Cell Ophthalmology Treatment Study (SCOTS) for Retina and Optic Nerve Disease: Case Report of Improvement in Relapsing Auto-Immune Optic Neuropathy. Neural Regeneration Research. 10;9:1507–1515, 2015.
- Weiss JN, Benes SC, Levy S. Stem Cell Ophthalmology Treatment Study (SCOTS): Improvement in Serpiginous Choroidopathy following Autologous Bone Marrow Derived Stem Cells. Neural Regeneration Research 11:1512–1516, 2016.
- Weiss JN, Benes SC, Levy S. Stem Cell Ophthalmology Treatment Study (SCOTS): Bone Marrow Derived Stem Cells in the Treatment of Leber Hereditary Optic Neuropathy. Neural Regeneration Research. 11:1685–1694, 2016.
- Weiss JN, Levy S. Neurologic Stem Cell Treatment Study (NEST) using bone marrow derived stem cells for the treatment of neurological disorders and injuries: study protocol for a nonrandomized efficacy trial. Clin Transl Degener Dis. 12;1(4):176–180, 2016.
- Weiss JN, Benes SC, Levy S. Stem Cell Ophthalmology Treatment Study: bone marrow derived stem cells in the treatment of non-arteritic ischemic optic neuropathy (NAION). Stem Cell Investigation. November 2017. http://sci.amegroups.com/issue/view/632.
- Weiss JN, Levy S. Autologous bone-marrow derived stem cells in the treatment of "untreatable" optic nerve and retinal conditions. EC Ophthalmology 9.5(2018):332–336.
- Weiss JN, Levy S. Stem Cell Ophthalmology Treatment Study: bone marrow derived stem cells in the treatment of Retinitis Pigmentosa. Stem Cell Investigation. http://dxb.doi.org/10.21037/sci.2018.04.02.
- Weiss JN, Levy S. Dynamic Light Scattering Spectroscopy of the Retina – A non-invasive quantitative technique to objectively document visual improvement following ocular stem cell treatment. Stem Cell Investig. 2019;6:8. https://doi.org/10.21037/sci.2019.03.01.
- Weiss JN, Levy S. Stem Cell Ophthalmology Treatment Study (SCOTS): Bone marrow derived stem cells in the treatment of Usher syndrome. Stem Cell Investig. 2019;9:9. https://doi.org/10.21037/sci.2019.08.07.
- Weiss JN, Levy S. Stem Cell Ophthalmology Treatment Study (SCOTS): Autologous bone-marrow derived stem cells in the treatment of hereditary macular degeneration. EC Ophthalmology 10.7 (2019): 536–542.
- Weiss JN, Levy S. Stem Cell Ophthalmology Treatment Study (SCOTS): Bone marrow derived stem cells in the treatment of Dominant Optic Atrophy. Stem Cell Investig. 2019; https://doi.org/10.21037/sci.2019.11.01.

- Weiss JN, Levy S. Stem Cell Ophthalmology Treatment Study (SCOTS): Bone marrow derived stem cells in the treatment of Age-related Macular Degeneration. Medicines 2020, 7,16. https://doi.org/10.3390/medicines7040016, 1–13.
- Weiss, JN, Levy, S. Stem Cell Ophthalmology Treatment Study (SCOTS): Bone Marrow-Derived Stem Cells in the Treatment of Stargardt Disease. Medicines 2021, 8, 10. https://doi.org/10.3390/medicines8020010, 1–10.

United States

Recruiting

A Study of the Safety and Tolerability of ASP7317 in Adults Who Are Losing Their Clear, Sharp Central Vision Due to Geographic Atrophy Secondary to Dry Age-Related Macular Degeneration

ClinicalTrials.gov ID NCT03178149

Sponsor Astellas Institute for Regenerative Medicine
Information provided by Astellas Pharma Inc (Astellas Institute for Regenerative Medicine) (Responsible Party)
Last Update Posted 2023-06-08

Study Overview

Brief Summary
This study is for adults 50 years or older who are losing their clear, sharp central vision. Central vision is needed to be able to read and drive a car. They have been diagnosed with dry age-related macular degeneration (called dry AMD). The macula is the center part of the back of the eye that allows you to see fine detail. In an advanced stage of this disease, areas of the macula die (atrophy), resulting in vision loss. This is called geographic atrophy. This study is looking at a new treatment called ASP7317. It is for slowing or reversing atrophy in dry AMD. ASP7317 is a specially created type of cells derived from human stem cells. ASP7317 cells are injected into the macula of the eye while the person is under anesthesia (local or general). An immunosuppressive medicine (tacrolimus) is also taken around the time of injection of the cells to prevent the body from rejecting them.

This study looks at how safe ASP7317 is at three different dose levels. Researchers want to learn if the different dose levels of ASP7317 work without causing unwanted medical problems. Each of the three doses will be given to two groups of people. The first group will be those who have severe vision loss. The second group will be those who have moderate vision loss. The doses are low, medium, and high numbers of cells. Tacrolimus will be taken by mouth for 34 days, starting around the time of the injection of ASP7317. In addition, medicines to prevent infection will be taken by mouth for up to 4 weeks starting around the time ASP7317 cells are injected.

Each week for the first 4 weeks after the ASP7317 cells have been injected, people taking part in the study will visit the clinic so the researchers can make assessments. Then they will visit again, at weeks 6, 8, 12, 16, 26, and 52 (the last week of the study).

A substudy will be available at some clinics. These clinics will use a special camera that will allow researchers to look at images of the macular atrophy over time.

Detailed Description
The study consists of the following periods: Screening (up to 45 days) and the Study Period (52 weeks post-treatment).

Official Title
A Phase 1b, Multicenter, Dose Escalation, Evaluation of Safety and Tolerability of ASP7317 for Geographic Atrophy Secondary to Age-related Macular Degeneration

Conditions
Age-Related Macular Degeneration

Intervention/Treatment
- Drug: ASP7317
- Drug: tacrolimus

Other Study ID Numbers
- 7317-CL-0003

Study Start (Actual)
2018-07-13

Primary Completion (Estimated)
2024-08-31

Study Completion (Estimated)
2024-08-31

Enrollment (Estimated)
18

Study Type
Interventional

Phase
Phase 1

Study Contact
Name: Astellas Institute for Regenerative Medicine
Phone Number: 800-888-7704
Email: astellas.registration@astellas.com
United States
Arizona Locations

Phoenix, Arizona, United States, 85053
Withdrawn
Retinal Consultants of Arizona LTD, Retinal Research Institute

California Locations

Los Angeles, California, United States, 90095
Recruiting
Jules Stein Eye Institute

Palo Alto, California, United States, 94303
Recruiting
Stanford University Byers Eye Institute

Florida Locations

Fort Myers, Florida, United States, 33912
Withdrawn
Retina Consultants of Southwest Florida & National Ophthalmic Research Institute

Pensacola, Florida, United States, 35203
Recruiting
Retina Specialty Institute

Georgia Locations

Atlanta, Georgia, United States, 30322
Recruiting
Emory University Eye Center

Massachusetts Locations

Boston, Massachusetts, United States, 02114
Withdrawn
Mass Eye and Ear Infirmary Ophthalmology Clinical Research Office

New Jersey Locations

New Brunswick, New Jersey, United States, 08901
Withdrawn
NJ Retina

Pennsylvania Locations

Philadelphia, Pennsylvania, United States, 19107
Recruiting
Mid-Atlantic Retina

Tennessee Locations

Nashville, Tennessee, United States, 37203
Recruiting
Tennessee Retina, PC

Texas Locations

McAllen, Texas, United States, 78503
Active, not recruiting
Valley Retina Institute

Washington Locations

Seattle, Washington, United States, 98104
Withdrawn
University of Washington

Eligibility Criteria
Description

General Inclusion Criteria

- Participant must be willing to take tacrolimus and willing to discontinue any medications that have a known strong interaction with tacrolimus.
- Participant is able and willing to undertake all scheduled visits and assessments up to the week 52 visit.
- Participant who is taking an antidepressant must be on a stable and effective dosage and must be willing to take it reliably for as long as it is required.
- Participant must be willing and medically suitable to undergo monitored anesthesia care during the vitrectomy and subretinal injection.
- Participant agrees not to participate in another interventional study until the 52-week visit has been completed.
- Female participant is not pregnant and at least one of the following conditions apply:
  - Not a woman of childbearing potential (WOCBP)
  - WOCBP who agrees to follow the contraceptive guidance from the time of informed consent through at least 52 weeks after investigational product (IP) administration.
- Female participant must agree not to breastfeed starting at screening and throughout the study period and for 52 weeks after IP administration.
- Female participant must not donate ova starting at first dose of IP and throughout the study period and for 52 weeks after IP administration.
- Male participant with female partner(s) of childbearing potential (including breastfeeding partner) must agree to use contraception throughout the treatment period and for 52 weeks after IP administration.
- Male participant must not donate sperm during the treatment period and for 52 weeks after IP administration.
- Male participant with pregnant partner(s) must agree to remain abstinent or use a condom for the duration of the pregnancy throughout the study period and for 52 weeks after IP administration.

Ocular Inclusion Criteria: Study Eye (Both Groups 1 and 2)

- Participant has bilateral geographic atrophy (GA) secondary to Age-Related Macular Degeneration (AMD). GA is defined as sharply demarcated areas of loss of the retinal pigment epithelial/epithelium (RPE).
- Participant has no evidence of prior or active choroidal neovascularization (CNV) with optical coherence tomography angiography (OCT-A) or indocyanine green angiography (ICG-A), as assessed by the reading center.
- Participant has the absence of exudation as assessed by fluorescein angiography (FA) and spectral domain-optical coherence tomography (SD-OCT).
- Participant has the presence of either banded or diffuse hyper autofluorescence in the junctional zone of GA as assessed by the central reading center.
- Participant has sufficiently clear ocular media, adequate pupillary dilation, and fixation to permit quality fundus imaging.
- Participant is willing to discontinue vitamins/supplements for AMD (e.g., Age-Related Eye Disease Study [AREDS] 2) at least 30 days before IP administration through 52 weeks after IP administration.
- Participant is pseudophakic.

Ocular Inclusion Criteria: Study Eye (Group 1 only)

- For Cohort 1, the participant has a BCVA between light perception and </= 23 Early Treatment Diabetic Retinopathy Study (ETDRS) letters at the screening visit. For Cohorts 2 and 3, the participant has a BCVA score between 20 (>/= 20/400) and 37 (</=20/200) ETDRS letters at the screening visit.
- Participant has the total GA area </= 30.5 mm^2 (</=12 disc areas [DA]).

Ocular Inclusion Criteria: Study Eye (Group 2 only)

- Participant has BCVA score between 38 (> 20/200) and 63 (</=20/63) ETDRS letters during the screening visit.
- Participant has a total GA area of >/= 5.1 mm^2 and < 17.8 mm^2 (>/=2 and </=7 DA, respectively) and must reside completely within the fundus autofluorescence (FAF) imaging field (Field 2–30 degree image centered on the fovea). If GA is multifocal, at least 1 focal lesion must be >/= 2.5 mm^2 (>/=1 DA).
- Participant has a difference in mean mesopic sensitivity </=2 dB between 2 tests at screening. If not </=2 dB, a third test may be conducted and mean values between the second and third assessments must be </=2 dB.

General Exclusion Criteria

- Participant has a history of recurrent varicella-zoster virus (VZV) infection or a clinical diagnosis of VZV infection within 4 weeks of the baseline visit.
- Participant has a history of recurrent cytomegalovirus (CMV) infection or a clinical diagnosis of CMV infection within 4 weeks of the baseline visit.
- Participant has a positive tuberculosis (TB) test during the screening period by an interferon-gamma release assay (e.g., QuantiFERON) within the 6 months prior to the screening. If a participant has tested negative for TB within the 6 months prior to the screening visit, retesting is not required unless clinically indicated.

- Participant has a history or suspected active infection of toxoplasmosis or presence of elevated immunoglobulin M (IgM) toxoplasmosis titer within 4 weeks of the baseline visit.
- Participant has an active infection (ocular or non-ocular) requiring the prolonged or chronic use of antimicrobial or anti-infective agents.
- Participant has a current malignancy or history of malignancy within the past 5 years, except non-metastatic basal or squamous cell carcinoma or keratoacanthoma or Bowen's disease or carcinoma in situ of the cervix that has been successfully treated.
- Participant has a history of a solid organ or bone marrow transplant.
- Participant had any condition that would prohibit the use of systemic immunosuppression with tacrolimus.
- Participant is receiving or has received any immunosuppressive therapy (IMT) (other than topical, inhaled, or low-dose systemic corticosteroid use not exceeding 7.5 mg of prednisone daily [or equivalent]) within 6 weeks or 5 plasma half-lives, whichever is longer, prior to the administration of adjunct study medications.
- Participant has a history of myocardial infarction in the previous 12 months and whose disease is either unstable and/or symptomatic (e.g., angina, dyspnea, etc.).
- Participant has electrocardiogram (ECG) results that are clinically significant and could either jeopardize the safety of the participant, impact the participant's ability to comply with the study visit schedule, or impact the validity of the study results. Participants with a mean Fridericia-corrected QT interval of > 430 ms (for males) and > 450 ms (for females) at screening must be cleared by a cardiologist prior to the baseline visit.
- Participant has a study day diastolic blood pressure > 95 mmHg, at either the screening or baseline visit. Study day blood pressure is defined as the average of the second and third readings at a study visit. If the study day blood pressure exceeds the limits, 1 additional triplicate can be taken.
- Participant has an estimated glomerular filtration rate (eGFR) of </= 45 mL/min, calculated by the chronic kidney disease epidemiology collaboration (CKD-EPI) equation.
- Participant has an alanine aminotransferase (ALT), aspartate aminotransferase (AST), or gamma-glutamyltransferase (GGT) and total bilirubin (TBL) >/= 2 times the upper limit of normal (ULN).
- Participant has severe anemia (hemoglobin < 9 g/dL [male] or hemoglobin < 8 g/dL [female]), leucopenia (white blood cell count <2500/mm^3), thrombocytopenia (platelet count <80000/mm^3), or polycythemia (hematocrit >54% [male] or hematocrit > 49% [female]).
- Participant has a hemoglobin A1c > 8.5%.
- Participant has a clinically significant coagulopathy (i.e., activated partial thromboplastin time [aPTT] >/= 1.5 times the ULN and/or prothrombin time adjusted for the international normalized ratio [PT-INR] >/=2.0).
- Participant has serology results indicative of having syphilis, Lyme disease, human immunodeficiency virus infection or active infection with hepatitis A

virus (HAV), hepatitis B virus (HBV), hepatitis C virus (HCV), or varicella-zoster virus (VZV).

- Participant has a history of familial adenomatous polyposis or inflammatory bowel disease (i.e., Crohn's disease, ulcerative colitis).
- Participant has a history of allergic reactions to mydriatics or fluorescein.
- Participant has a history of gene therapy or cell transplant therapy, including ASP7316, in a prior clinical study.
- Participant has participated in any studies of an investigational drug (excluding vitamins and minerals for AMD studies) within 12 weeks prior to the screening visit.
- Participant is unwilling to discontinue or avoid any CYP3A4 inducers (e.g., rifampin, rifabutin, phenytoin, carbamazepine, phenobarbital, St John's Wort) or participant is unwilling to discontinue or avoid protease inhibitors (e.g., nelfinavir, telaprevir, boceprevir), direct Factor Xa inhibitors, direct thrombin inhibitors, verapamil, diltiazem, or erythromycin while taking tacrolimus.
- Participant has a positive urine screen for drugs of abuse (amphetamines, barbiturates, benzodiazepines, opiates, cocaine, phencyclidine, and methadone) unless the drug is taken for a documented medical condition and under the supervision of a physician.

Ocular Exclusion Criteria: Study Eye

- Participant has macular degeneration due to causes other than AMD (e.g., Stargardt disease, cone–rod dystrophy, toxic maculopathies, etc.)
- Participant has foveal sparing as determined by the presence of potentially viable photoreceptors, as evidenced by the presence of ellipsoid zone (EZ) </= 250 microns from the foveal center, based on reading center assessments at the screening visit.
- Participant has a history of vitrectomy or submacular surgery or any surgical intervention for AMD.
- Participant has prior treatment with photodynamic therapy (e.g., Visudyne®), intraocular external-beam radiation therapy, or transpupillary thermotherapy.
- Participant has a history of previous laser photocoagulation for choroidal neovascularization (CNV), diabetic macular edema, retinal vein occlusion, and proliferative diabetic retinopathy.
- Participant has a history of intravitreal drug delivery (e.g., anti-VEGF drugs, anti-complement agents, intravitreal corticosteroid injection, or device implantation) within 1 year prior to the screening visit.
- Participant has an abnormality of the vitreoretinal interface (e.g., tractional epiretinal membrane), which can interfere with the measurement of macular thickness or with the potential for macular structural damage.
- Participant has a history of cystoid macular edema, retinal vascular occlusion, central serous chorioretinopathy, macular hole, or retinoschisis.

- Participant has active or history of intraocular inflammation such as uveitis, chorioretinitis, and optic neuropathy.
- Participant has the presence of an ocular toxoplasmosis scar.
- Participant has nevus of Ota (oculodermal melanocytosis), a pigmented choroidal lesion showing characteristics associated with a high risk of malignancy (e.g., elevated lesion), or a choroidal nevus in the macula.
- Participant has pathologic myopia defined as a spherical equivalent of > 8.00 diopters or axial length > 28 mm at the screening visit, or myopic macular degeneration or posterior staphyloma.
- Participant has glaucoma with uncontrolled intraocular pressure (IOP) (defined as IOP > 30 mmHg despite treatment with anti-glaucoma medication) or is using more than two agents to control IOP or a history of glaucoma-filtering surgery.
- Participant has a history of corneal transplantation.
- Participant has a monocular vision; no light perception in the fellow eye or anophthalmic in the fellow eye.
- Participant has a contraindication to pupil dilation.
- Participant has any other ocular condition that can interfere with the assessment of imaging data.
- ADAPTIVE OPTICS RETINAL IMAGING SUBSTUDY ONLY: Either eye with GA area >/=7 DA, or has photosensitivity, or is at high risk for light hazard, or has a multifocal intraocular lens, or has an optical zone < 5 mm in diameter, or has capsulorhexis smaller than 5 mm. Note: this is not an exclusion criterion for the participant from the study, but only an exclusion of the participant's eye(s) from the Adaptive Optics Retinal Imaging substudy.

Ages Eligible for Study
50 Years and older (Adult, Older Adult)

Sexes Eligible for Study
All

Accepts Healthy Volunteers
No
Study Plan

Design Details
Primary Purpose: Treatment
Allocation: Non-Randomized
Interventional Model: Sequential Assignment
Masking: None (Open Label)

Arms and interventions

Participant group/arm	Intervention/treatment
Experimental: ASP7317 Dose Escalation (Group 1) Group 1 will consist of participants with Severe Vision Impairment. Successive cohorts of participants (three participants/cohort) will be treated in each escalating dose cohort (cohort 1: low cells/dose; cohort 2: medium cells/dose; cohort 3: high cells/dose). Sentinel dosing will be required for each dose level. After the first participant in Group 1 dose cohort is dosed and followed for 3 weeks, the independent Data Safety Monitoring Board (DSMB) will review the three-week safety data and recommend if the second and third participants in Group 1 dose cohort may be treated. The DSMB recommendation to progress to the next dosing cohort will be based on three-week follow-up safety review of the second and third participants in the preceding dose cohort. Participants will receive tacrolimus twice daily starting at baseline through week 4.	Drug: ASP7317 • Subretinal injection Drug: tacrolimus • Oral • Other Names: – FK506 – Prograf®
Experimental: ASP7317 Dose Escalation (Group 2) Group 2 will consist of participants with Moderate Vision Impairment. Successive cohorts of participants (three participants/cohort) will be treated in each escalating dose cohort (cohort 4: low cells/dose; cohort 5: medium cells/dose; cohort 6: high cells/dose). Dosing in cohort 4 (low cells/dose) may commence following the DSMB recommendation to begin dosing in Group 1 cohort 2 (medium cells/dose). Dosing in Group 2 cohort 5 (medium cells/dose) may commence following DSMB review of the three-week safety data of the first participant in Group 1 cohort 2 (medium cells/dose). Similarly, dosing in Group 2 cohort 6 (high cells/dose) may commence following DSMB review of three-week safety data of the first participant in Group 1 cohort 3 (high cells/dose). Participants will receive tacrolimus twice daily starting at baseline through week 4	Drug: ASP7317 • Subretinal injection Drug: tacrolimus • Oral • Other Names: – FK506 – Prograf®

Primary outcome measures

Outcome measure	Measure description	Time frame
Safety as assessed by incidence, frequency, and severity of treatment-emergent adverse events (TEAES)	Adverse events (AEs) will be coded using Medical Dictionary for Regulatory Activities (MedDRA). An Adverse Event is any untoward medical occurrence in a patient or clinical study participant, temporally associated with the use of ASP7317, the adjunct study medications and the study procedures, whether or not considered related to ASP7317, the adjunct study medications and the study procedures A Treatment Emergent Adverse Event (TEAE) is defined as an AE beginning or worsening in severity after starting administration of the adjunct study medication	Up to 52 Weeks
Safety as assessed by incidence, frequency and severity of Serious Adverse Events (SAEs)	An SAE is defined as any untoward medical occurrence that, at any dose: results in death; is life-threatening; requires inpatient hospitalization or prolongation of existing hospitalization; results in persistent or significant disability/incapacity; results in congenital anomaly or birth defect or other medically important events	Up to 52 Weeks

Safety assessed by Adverse Events (AEs) of special interest	AEs of special interest include: ectopic or proliferative cell growth (retinal pigment epithelial/epithelium (RPE) or non-RPE) with adverse clinical consequence; any new diagnosis of an immune-mediated disorder; any new cancer, irrespective of prior history; unexpected, clinically significant AEs possibly related to the cell transplant procedure; immunosuppressive therapy (IMT) or ASP7317 (e.g., graft failure or rejection)	Up to 52 Weeks
Number of participants with cellular graft failure or rejection	Evidence of cellular graft failure or rejection will be assessed by best-corrected visual acuity (BCVA), slit lamp examination, dilated indirect ophthalmoscopy, fundus photographs, spectral domain-optical coherence tomography (SD-OCT), and fluorescein angiography (FA), when performed	Up to 52 Weeks
Incidence of cellular graft failure or rejection	Evidence of cellular graft failure or rejection will be assessed by best-corrected visual acuity (BCVA), slit lamp examination, dilated indirect ophthalmoscopy, fundus photographs, spectral domain-optical coherence tomography (SD-OCT), and fluorescein angiography (FA) when performed	Up to 52 Weeks

Secondary outcome measures

Outcome measure	Measure description	Time frame
Mean change from baseline in area of Geographic Atrophy (GA) (mm^2) in the study eye and fellow eye	GA will be measured by blue-light and near-infrared fundus autofluorescence (NIR FAF) (definitely decreased autofluorescence (DDAF)) and spectral domain-optical coherence tomography (SD-OCT) (area of ellipsoid zone (EZ) defect, area of outer nuclear layer (ONL) defect)	Baseline, Weeks 26 and 52/End of Study (EOS)
Mean percent change from baseline in area of Geographic Atrophy (GA) (mm^2) in study eye and fellow eye	GA will be measured by blue-light and near-infrared fundus autofluorescence (NIR FAF) (definitely decreased autofluorescence (DDAF)) and spectral domain-optical coherence tomography (SD-OCT) (area of ellipsoid zone (EZ) defect, area of outer nuclear layer (ONL) defect)	Baseline, Weeks 26 and 52/End of Study (EOS)
Mean change from baseline in the square root transformation of Geographic Atrophy (GA) area in the study eye and fellow eye	GA will be measured by blue-light and near-infrared fundus autofluorescence (NIR FAF) (definitely decreased autofluorescence (DDAF)) and spectral domain-optical coherence tomography (SD-OCT) (area of ellipsoid zone (EZ) defect, area of outer nuclear layer (ONL) defect)	Baseline, Weeks 26 and 52/End of Study (EOS)
Mean change from baseline in best-corrected visual acuity (BCVA) score in study eye and fellow eye	BCVA will be measured by an assessor certified to use the Early Treatment of Diabetic Retinopathy Study (ETDRS) method. The BCVA score (in letter units) will be reported	Baseline, Weeks 1, 4, 6, 8, 12, 16, 26 and 52/ End of Study (EOS)

Sponsor
Astellas Institute for Regenerative Medicine

Collaborators
No information provided

Investigators
- Study Director: Medical Director, Astellas Institute for Regenerative Medicine

General Publications
No publications available

Caribbean

Recruiting

Safety of Cultured Allogeneic Adult Umbilical Cord Derived Mesenchymal Stem Cells for Eye Diseases

ClinicalTrials.gov ID NCT05147701

Sponsor The Foundation for Orthopaedics and Regenerative Medicine
Information provided by The Foundation for Orthopaedics and Regenerative Medicine (Responsible Party)
Last Update Posted 2022-10-27

Study Overview

Brief Summary
This trial will study the safety and efficacy of intravenous and sub-tenon delivery of cultured allogeneic adult umbilical cord derived mesenchymal stem cells for the treatment of Eye diseases

Detailed Description
This patient-funded trial aims to study the safety and efficacy of intravenous and sub-tenon delivery of cultured allogeneic adult umbilical cord derived mesenchymal stem cells (UC-MSCs) for the treatment of Eye Diseases. The total dose will be 100 million cells. Patients will be evaluated within one month pretreatment and at 1, 6, 12, 24, 36, and 48 months post-treatment for safety and efficacy.

For patients with more severe disease an autologous Effector cells (activated lymphocytes) treatment will be utilized created from the patient's own cells obtained by apheresis.

Official Title
Safety of Cultured Allogeneic Adult Umbilical Cord Derived Mesenchymal Stem Cells for the Treatment of Eye Diseases

Conditions
Eye Diseases
Retinitis Pigmentosa
Glaucoma
Diabetic Retinopathy
Macular Degeneration
Traumatic Optic Neuropathy
Optic Atrophy

Intervention/Treatment
- Biological: AlloRx

Other Study ID Numbers
- ATG-1-MSC-014

Study Start (Actual)
2022-02-01

Primary Completion (Estimated)
2026-01

Study Completion (Estimated)
2026-01

Enrollment (Estimated)
20

Study Type
Interventional

Phase
Phase 1

Antigua and Barbuda

St. John's, Antigua and Barbuda
Recruiting
Medical Surgical Associates Center

Contact
Chadwick Prodromos, M.D.
8476996810 care@thepsci.com

Argentina

Buenos Aires, Argentina
Recruiting
Center for Investigation in Tissue Engineering and Cellular Therapy

Contact
Chadwick Prodromos, M.D.
8476996810 ext 202 Care@thepsci.com

Mexico
N.L Locations

San Pedro Garza García, N.L, Mexico
Recruiting
Medyca Bosques

Contact
Chadwick Prodromos, M.D.
8476996810 ext 202 Care@thepsci.com

Eligibility Criteria
Description

Inclusion Criteria
- Diagnosis of eye disease
- Understanding and willingness to sign a written informed consent document

Exclusion Criteria
- Active infection
- Active cancer
- Chronic multisystem organ failure
- Pregnancy
- Clinically significant Abnormalities on pre-treatment laboratory evaluation
- Medical condition that would (based on the opinion of the investigator) compromise patient's safety
- Continued drug abuse
- Pre-menopausal women not using contraception
- Previous organ transplant
- Hypersensitivity to sulfur

Ages Eligible for Study
(Child, Adult, Older Adult)

Sexes Eligible for Study
All

Accepts Healthy Volunteers
No

Design Details
Primary Purpose: Treatment
Allocation: N/A
Interventional Model: Single Group Assignment
Masking: None (Open Label)

Arms and interventions

Participant group/arm	Intervention/treatment
Experimental: Treatment Group (AlloRx) intravenous and sub-tenon delivery (total dose of 100 million cells)	Biological: AlloRx • Cultured allogeneic adult umbilical cord derived mesenchymal stem cells

Primary outcome measures

Outcome measure	Measure description	Time frame
Safety (adverse events)	Clinical monitoring of possible adverse events or complications	Four year follow-up

Sponsor
The Foundation for Orthopaedics and Regenerative Medicine

Collaborators
No information provided

Investigators
- Principal Investigator: Chadwick Prodromos, MD, The Foundation for Orthopaedics and Regenerative Medicine

General Publications
- Sung Y, Lee SM, Park M, Choi HJ, Kang S, Choi BI, Lew H. Treatment of traumatic optic neuropathy using human placenta-derived mesenchymal stem cells in Asian patients. Regen Med. 2020 Oct;15(10):2163–2179. https://doi.org/10.2217/rme-2020-0044. Epub 2020 Dec 14.
- Zhao T, Liang Q, Meng X, Duan P, Wang F, Li S, Liu Y, Yin ZQ. Intravenous Infusion of Umbilical Cord Mesenchymal Stem Cells Maintains and Partially Improves Visual Function in Patients with Advanced Retinitis Pigmentosa. Stem Cells Dev. 2020 Aug;29(16):1029–1037. https://doi.org/10.1089/scd.2020.0037. Epub 2020 Jul 15.
- Ozmert E, Arslan U. Management of retinitis pigmentosa by Wharton's jelly derived mesenchymal stem cells: preliminary clinical results. Stem Cell Res Ther. 2020 Jan 13;11(1):25. https://doi.org/10.1186/s13287-020-1549-6.

China

Not Yet Recruiting

Preparation of Patient Autologous-Induced Pluripotent Stem Cell-Derived Retinal Cells for AMD

ClinicalTrials.gov ID NCT05991986

Sponsor Zhongshan Ophthalmic Center, Sun Yat-Sen University
Information provided by Xiufeng Zhong, Zhongshan Ophthalmic Center, Sun Yat-Sen University (Responsible Party)
Last Update Posted 2023-08-15

Study Overview

Brief Summary

This project intends to collect participant somatic cells to prepare autologous-induced pluripotent stem cell-derived retinal cells for future cell therapy of age-related macular degeneration patient.

Detailed Description

One or more types of somatic cells will be collected from every participant by collecting approximately 100–500 ml of midstream urine, 20–30 ml of peripheral blood, skin biopsies (3 mm), conjunctival biopsies (5 mm × 5 mm), etc. Then, these somatic cells will be used to prepare patient autologous induced pluripotent stem cell-derived retinal cells for the cell therapy of age-related macular degeneration patient.

Official Title

Production of Patient Autologous Induced Pluripotent Stem Cell-derived Retinal Cells for Age-Related Macular Degeneration

Conditions

Age-Related Macular Degeneration

Intervention/Treatment

- Other: somatic cell collection

Other Study ID Numbers

- 2023KYPJ224

Study Start (Estimated)

2023-08

Primary Completion (Estimated)

2026-07-31

Study Completion (Estimated)

2026-07-31

Enrollment (Estimated)

10

Study Type

Observational

Study Contact

Name: Wenjing Yin
Phone Number: 020-87330290
Email: wenjingyina@163.com
No location data

Eligibility Criteria
Description

Inclusion Criteria

- Aged 55–80 years
- Clinical diagnosis is consistent with the definition of advanced age-related macular degeneration
- The BCVA of the target eye will be lower than 20/200
- -8.00 D < refraction < +8.00 D, 21 mm < anteroposterior axis ≤ 28 mm
- Voluntary as test subjects, informed consent, regular follow-up on time
- Voluntary as test subjects to join the associated clinical research on autologous iPSC-derived retinal cell therapy for AMD (ethical approval and informed consent documents will be applied and signed separately)

Exclusion Criteria

- Macular atrophy caused by other diseases in addition to AMD
- Malignant tumor and history of malignancy
- Any immune deficiency
- Lens opacities (affecting the central vision), glaucoma, uveitis, retinal detachment, inherited retinal dystrophy, optic neuropathy, and other ocular histories
- Other intraocular surgery histories besides cataract surgery
- Severe heart failure or the left ventricular ejection fraction <35% in the previous 6 months
- Dialysis or eGFR <20 ml/min/1.73 m^2
- Urine protein/urine creatinine ratio ≥ 1 g/g
- Creatinine or albumin/urine creatinine ratio ≥ 600 mg/g
- Chronic liver disease with ALT three times over the upper limit of normal value
- Combined with severe systemic diseases, such as heart failure, liver disease, COPD, etc.
- Combined with severe infectious diseases, such as HIV, HBV, HCV, syphilis, etc.
- HCV-RNA positive, HBV-DNA >103 IU/ml, or TB, etc., during the infectious period
- Use anticoagulant, or the platelet function is still not restored to normal after stopping antiplatelet drugs for 10 days
- Abnormal blood coagulation function or other laboratory tests
- Use glucocorticoids, immunosuppressive drugs, or antipsychotic drugs in the previous 3 months
- Use antipsychotic drugs in the previous 3 months, such as antidepressants drugs and antimanic drugs;
- Allergy to tacrolimus or other macrolides
- A history of addiction to alcoholism or prohibited drugs
- Be participating in other intervention clinical trials or receiving other study medications
- Informed refusal
- Some other situations which might increase the risks of the subjects or interfere with clinical trials, such as mental disorders and cognitive dysfunction

Study Population
AMD patients

Ages Eligible for Study
55 Years to 80 Years (Adult, Older Adult)

Sexes Eligible for Study
All

Accepts Healthy Volunteers
No

Sampling Method
Non-Probability Sample

Design Details
Observational Model: Other
Time Perspective: Other
Biospecimen Retention: Samples with DNA
Biospecimen Description: somatic cells isolated from urine, peripheral blood, skin biopsies, conjunctiva biopsies, etc.

Cohorts and interventions

Intervention/treatment
Other: somatic cell collection • One or more types of somatic cells will be collected from every participant by collecting approximately 100–500 ml of midstream urine, 20–30 ml of peripheral blood, skin biopsies (3 mm), conjunctiva biopsies (5 mm × 5 mm), etc.

Primary outcome measures

Outcome measure	Measure description	Time frame
Somatic cell collection	Somatic cell collection	2023.8.1 ~ 2026.7.31

Sponsor
Zhongshan Ophthalmic Center, Sun Yat-Sen University

Collaborators
No information provided

Investigators
- Study Director: Xiufeng Zhong, Doctor Zhongshan Ophthalmic Center, Sun Yat-Sen University

General Publications
No publications available

China

Recruiting

Safety and Efficacy of Autologous Transplantation of iPSC-RPE in the Treatment of Macular Degeneration

ClinicalTrials.gov ID NCT05445063

Sponsor Beijing Tongren Hospital
Information provided by Beijing Tongren Hospital (Responsible Party)
Last Update Posted 2022-07-06

Study Overview

Brief Summary
This project intends to perform autologous transplantation of induced pluripotent stem cell-derived retinal pigment epithelium (iPSC-RPE). The clinical-grade RPE will be transplanted into subretinal space to treat refractory age-related macular degeneration. The efficacy and safety of RPE transplants to treat macular degeneration will be monitored and analyzed with results from EDTRS, BCVA, OCT, ERG, microperimetry, and fluorescein angiography, before and after the treatment.

Detailed Description
The investigators will generate iPSC lines from recruited participants and differentiate the iPSC into RPE. Autologous iPSC-derived RPE will be transplanted into participants eyes by subretinal injections. The safety and efficacy will be closely monitored and analyzed.

Official Title
Safety and Efficacy of Autologous Transplantation of Induced Pluripotent Stem Cell-Derived Retinal Pigment Epithelium in the Treatment of Macular Degeneration

Conditions
Macular Degeneration

Intervention/Treatment
- Biological: Autologous iPSC-derived RPE

Other Study ID Numbers
- 2021-214

Study Start (Estimated)
2022-08

Primary Completion (Estimated)
2026-07

Study Completion (Estimated)
2026-12

Enrollment (Estimated)
10

Study Type
Interventional

Phase
Phase 1

Study Contact
Name: Xiaohui Zhang
Phone Number: +0086-(010)58265915
Email: zhangxh711@126.com
China
Beijing Locations

Beijing, Beijing, China, 100730
Recruiting
Beijing Tongren Hospital, Capital Medical University

Contact
Zi-Bing Jin, Doctor
+0086-(010)58265913 jinzibing@foxmail.com

Eligibility Criteria
Description

Inclusion Criteria
- Aged 50–75 years
- Clinical diagnosis is consistent with the definition of late dry AMD in the age-related eye disease study (AREDS), with one or more >250 μm geographic atrophy in the fovea
- Clinical diagnosis is wet AMD, but no obvious efficacy after conventional treatment
- The BCVA of the target eye will be 0.05–0.3
- Voluntary as test subjects, informed consent, regular follow-up on time

Exclusion Criteria
- One-eyed subjects
- Macular atrophy caused by other diseases in addition to AMD
- Suffer from retinitis pigmentosa, choroidal retinitis, central serous choroiditis, diabetic retinopathy, or other retinal vascular and degenerative diseases besides AMD
- Lens opacities (affecting the central vision), glaucoma, uveitis, retinal detachment, optic neuropathy, and other ocular histories

- Other intraocular surgery histories besides cataract surgery
- Combined with severe systemic diseases, such as heart failure, liver disease, renal insufficiency, cor pulmonale, and COPD in the previous 12 months
- Combined with severe infectious diseases, such as HIV, HBV, HCV, syphilis, and tuberculosis;
- Abnormal blood coagulation function or other laboratory tests
- If female and of childbearing potential, pregnant, breastfeeding, or planning to become pregnant through the study
- If the male refuses to use barrier and spermicide contraception during the study
- Malignant tumor and history of malignancy
- Any immune deficiency
- Allergy to tacrolimus or other macrolides
- Any immune deficiency
- Use glucocorticoids, immunosuppressive drugs, or antipsychotic drugs in the previous 3 months
- Use anticoagulant, or the platelet function is still not restored to normal after stopping antiplatelet drugs for 10 days
- A history of addiction to alcoholism or prohibited drugs
- Be participating in other intervention clinical trials or receiving other study medications
- Poor compliance, difficulty in completing the study, or refusal to informed consent
- Some other situations which might increase the risks of the subjects or interfere with clinical trials, such as mental disorders and cognitive dysfunction.

Ages Eligible for Study
50 Years to 75 Years (Adult, Older Adult)

Sexes Eligible for Study
All

Accepts Healthy Volunteers
No

Design Details
Primary Purpose: Treatment
Allocation: N/A
Interventional Model: Single Group Assignment
Masking: None (Open Label)

Arms and interventions

Participant group/arm	Intervention/treatment
Experimental: Participants receiving intervention Participants will receive autologous transplantation of induced pluripotent stem cell-derived retinal pigment epitheliums	Biological: Autologous iPSC-derived RPE • Autologous transplantation of iPSC-derived RPE

Primary outcome measures

Outcome measure	Measure description	Time frame
Safety measure	Safety will be assessed by Adverse Events (AEs) of special interest in regard to the investigational product. This will include obtaining information about Serious Adverse Events (SAEs) that are neurologic, infectious, hematologic or fatal, any AE that causes the subject to withdraw from the study, any new diagnosis of an ocular or immune-mediated disorder, cancer (irrespective of prior history), ectopic or proliferative cell growth (RPE or non-RPE) with adverse clinical consequence, unexpected, clinically significant AE possibly related to the cell transplant procedure or the investigational product (autologous iPSC-RPE), pregnancy in a female subject or the partner of a male subject and pregnancy outcome	12 months

Secondary Outcome Measures

Outcome measure	Measure description	Time frame
Best Corrected Visual Acuity (BCVA)	Change in visual acuity will be measured by an Early Treatment Diabetic Retinopathy Study (ETDRS) chart	12 months
Optical coherence tomography (OCT) imaging	The number of patients with serious retinal detachment, retinal hemorrhage, and cystoid macular edema, and the change in target treatment areas	12 months
Color and autofluorescence imaging	Change in target treatment areas	12 months
Fluorescein angiography	Change in target treatment areas	12 months
Fundus autofluorescence	Change in target treatment areas	12 months
Microperimetry	Exploratory evaluations for the change of retinal sensitivity from baseline in the region of interest	12 months
Electroretinography (ERG)	Exploratory evaluations for the change of retinal electrophysiology responses from baseline	12 months

Sponsor
Beijing Tongren Hospital

Collaborators
No information provided

Investigators
No information provided

General Publications
No publications available

Great Britain

Recruiting

A Study of Implantation of Retinal Pigment Epithelium in Subjects with Acute Wet Age-Related Macular Degeneration

ClinicalTrials.gov ID NCT01691261

Sponsor Moorfields Eye Hospital NHS Foundation Trust
Information provided by Moorfields Eye Hospital NHS Foundation Trust (Responsible Party)
Last Update Posted 2022-08-22

Study Overview

Brief Summary
Phase 1 trial of retinal pigment epithelium replacement in subjects with wet age-related macular degeneration in whom there is rapidly progressing vision loss.

Detailed Description
Phase 1, Open-Label, Safety and Feasibility Study of Implantation of PF-05206388 (human embryonic stem cell-derived retinal pigment epithelium) in subjects with wet age-related macular degeneration and rapid vision loss.

Official Title
Phase 1, Open-Label, Safety and Feasibility Study of Implantation of Pf-05206388 (Human Embryonic Stem Cell-Derived Retinal Pigment Epithelium (Rpe) Living Tissue Equivalent) in Subjects With Acute Wet Age-Related Macular Degeneration and Recent Rapid Vision Decline

Conditions
Age-Related Macular Degeneration

Intervention/Treatment
- Biological: PF-05206388

Other Study ID Numbers
- B4711001
- 2011-005493-37 (EudraCT Number)

Study Start (Actual)
2021-10-14

Primary Completion (Estimated)
2023-10-10

Study Completion (Estimated)
2024-03-14

Enrollment (Estimated)
10

Study Type
Interventional

Phase
Phase 1

Study Contact
Name: Tania West
Phone Number: 02072533411 ext 2036
Email: moorfields.resadmin@nhs.net

Study Contact Backup
Name: Daniela Narvaez
Phone Number: 02072533411 ext 2036
Email: moorfields.resadmin@nhs.net
United Kingdom

London, United Kingdom, EC1V 2PD
Recruiting
Moorfields Eye Hospital NHS Foundation Trust

London, United Kingdom, EC1V 2PD
Recruiting
Moorfields Eye Hospital NHS Foundation Trust

Contact
Moorfields R&D
020 7253 3411 ext 2937 moorfields.resadmin@nhs.net

Description

Inclusion Criteria
- Male and/or post-menopausal female subjects aged 60 years or above
- Diagnosis of wet Age-Related Macular Degeneration (AMD) plus rapid recent vision decline
- An informed consent document signed and dated by the subject or a legal representative

Exclusion Criteria
- Pregnant females; breastfeeding females; and females of childbearing potential
- Treatment with an investigational drug within 30 days (or as determined by the local requirement, whichever is longer) or five half-lives preceding the first dose of study medication
- Current or previous significant other ocular disease in the study eye, as determined by the investigator

Ages Eligible for Study
60 Years and older (Adult, Older Adult)

Sexes Eligible for Study
All

Accepts Healthy Volunteers
No

Design Details
Primary Purpose: Treatment
Allocation: N/A
Interventional Model: Single Group Assignment
Masking: None (open-label)

Arms and interventions

Participant group/arm	Intervention/treatment
Experimental: Treatment PF-05206388 Retinal Pigment Epithelium living tissue equivalent for intraocular use in the form of a monolayer of Retinal Pigmented Epithelial (RPE) cells immobilized on a polyester membrane	Biological: PF-05206388 • PF-05206388 will be provided as a Retinal Pigment Epithelium living tissue equivalent for intraocular use in the form of a monolayer of Retinal Pigmented Epithelial (RPE) cells immobilized on a polyester membrane. The membrane is approximately 6 mm × 3 mm and will contain a confluent layer of RPE cells, at a nominal dose of 17 mm^2. The implant is intended to be life-long

Primary outcome measures

Outcome measure	Measure description	Time frame
Incidence and severity of adverse events	The number of Adverse Events (AE) and Serious Adverse Events (SAE) noted during the study and an assessment of whether they are trial product related	52 weeks
Change in baseline in ETDRS best-corrected visual acuity (BCVA)—Proportion of subjects with an improvement of 15 letters or more at Week 24	The number of patients with a difference between the baseline BCVA and BCVA at 24 weeks in ETDRS letters, where the difference is 15 letters or more, as a percentage of the total number of cases	24 weeks

Secondary outcome measures

Outcome measure	Measure description	Time frame
Change in baseline in ETDRS best-corrected visual acuity (BCVA)—Proportion of subjects with an improvement of 15 letters or more	The number of patients with a difference between the baseline BCVA and BCVA at weeks 1, 2, 4, 8, 12, 16, 36, 52 in ETDRS letters, where the difference is 15 letters or more, as a percentage of the total number of cases	Weeks 1, 2, 4, 8, 12, 16, 36, 52
Mean change of best-corrected visual acuity (BCVA) from baseline by study visit	The mean difference between the baseline BCVA and final BCVA in ETDRS letters for all cases	52 weeks

Position of PF-05206388 by serial biomicroscopic evaluation	Measurement of movement in millimeters and rotation in degrees measure relative to baseline, at day 2 and weeks 1, 2, 4, 8, 10, 12, 16, 24, 36, and 52	Day 2 and Weeks 1, 2, 4, 8, 10, 12, 16, 24, 36, 52
Position and presence of pigmented RPE cells by serial fundus photography	The subjective reporting of the area of pigmentation as a % with cross-reference to the OCT at weeks 2, 4, 8, 10, 12, 16, 24, 36, and 52	Weeks 2, 4, 8, 10, 12, 16, 24, 36, 52
Mean change from baseline in contrast sensitivity by Pelli Robson test	The mean difference between the baseline BCVA and final BCVA in Pelli Robson letters read, across all subjects	Weeks 24, 52
Change in liver and renal function by blood tests and liver ultrasound	Record of any abnormalities in liver and renal function on blood testing and any abnormalities detected on the liver ultrasound	Weeks 24 and 52
Change in leakage or perfusion in normal fundal vasculature and presence of abnormal vasculature by fundus fluorescein angiography	Assessment and noting of abnormalities on Fundus fluorescein angiography at weeks 4, 8, 12, 24, and 52	Weeks 4, 8, 12, 24, and 52
Change in central 30 degree of visual function by Humphrey Field test	Recording and reporting of any changes on the central 30-degree field on the automated Humphrey Field test at weeks 4, 8, 12, 24, and 52	Weeks 4, 8, 12, 24, and 52
Change in thickness of RPE layer by B-mode orbital ultrasound	Recording of any changes in the thickness of the RPE layer by B-mode orbital ultrasound carried out by the ocular oncologist or medical physicist at weeks 4, 8, 16, 24, 36, and 52	Weeks 4, 8, 16, 24, 36, 52

Sponsor
Moorfields Eye Hospital NHS Foundation Trust

Collaborators
University College, London

Investigators
Study Director: Moorfields, Moorfields Eye Hospital NHS Foundation Trust

General Publications
No publications available

Great Britain

Not Yet Recruiting

Retinal Pigment Epithelium Safety Study for Patients in B4711001

ClinicalTrials.gov ID NCT03102138

Sponsor Moorfields Eye Hospital NHS Foundation Trust
Information provided by Moorfields Eye Hospital NHS Foundation Trust (Responsible Party)
Last Update Posted 2023-03-16

Study Overview

Brief Summary
This is a safety follow-up study. Patients enrolled in B4711001 will be followed for a further 4 years with regular visits to assess safety.

Official Title
Long-Term, Open-Label, Safety Follow-Up Study Following Transplantation Of Pf-05206388 (Human Embryonic Stem Cell-Derived Retinal Pigment Epithelium (RPE)) in Subjects with Acute Wet Age-Related Macular Degeneration and Recent Rapid Vision Decline

Conditions
Age-Related Macular Degeneration

Intervention/Treatment

Other Study ID Numbers
- B4711005
- 2015-002267-42 (EudraCT Number)

Study Start (Estimated)
2023-05-21

Primary Completion (Estimated)
2033-05-30

Study Completion (Estimated)
2033-05-30

Enrollment (Estimated)
10

Study Type
Observational

Study Contact
Name: Declan Flanagan
Phone Number: 07872414988
Email: moorfields.resadmin@nhs.net
United Kingdom

London, United Kingdom, EC1V 2PD
Moorfields Eye Hospital NHS Foundation Trust, 162 City Road

Eligibility Criteria
Description

Inclusion Criteria
- Evidence of a personally signed and dated informed consent document indicating that the subject has been informed of all pertinent aspects of the study
- Previous participation in Protocol B4711001 and received treatment with PF-05206388
- Subjects who are willing and able to comply with scheduled visits and study procedures

Exclusion Criteria
- there are no exclusion criteria

Study Population
Patients with AMD treated in main study

Ages Eligible for Study
60 Years and older (Adult, Older Adult)

Sexes Eligible for Study
All

Accepts Healthy Volunteers
No

Sampling Method
Non-Probability Sample

Design Details
Observational Model: Cohort
Time Perspective: Prospective

Cohorts and interventions

Group/cohort
Observation Subjects treated in B4711001 with PF-05206388 will be assessed

Primary outcome measures

Outcome measure	Measure description	Time frame
Incidence of serious adverse events and ocular adverse events	Incidence of serious adverse events and ocular adverse events will be monitored	4 years

Secondary outcome measures

Outcome measure	Measure description	Time frame
Change from baseline (pre-implantation) in ETDRS (Early Treatment of Diabetic Retinopathy Study) best-corrected visual acuity (BCVA)	Change from baseline (pre-implantation) in ETDRS (Early Treatment of Diabetic Retinopathy Study) best-corrected visual acuity (BCVA). The Proportion of subjects with an improvement of 15 letters or more at all time points will be assessed	4 years
Mean ETDRS BCVA and change from baseline (pre-implantation) at all time points	Mean ETDRS BCVA and change from baseline (pre-implantation) at all time points will be assessed	4 years

Sponsor
Moorfields Eye Hospital NHS Foundation Trust

Collaborators
No information provided

Investigators
- Principal Investigator: Lyndon da Cruz, Moorfields Eye Hospital NHS Foundation Trust

General Publications
No publications available

Chapter 4
Gene Therapy Trials

United States

Not Yet Recruiting

Phase I/II Study of SKG0106 Intraocular Solution in Patients with Neovascular Age-Related Macular Degeneration (nAMD)

ClinicalTrials.gov ID NCT05986864

Sponsor Skyline Therapeutics (US) Inc.
Information provided by Skyline Therapeutics (Skyline Therapeutics (US) Inc.) (Responsible Party)
Last Update Posted 2023-09-28

Study Overview

Brief Summary
This is a phase 1/2 clinical study to evaluate the safety, preliminary efficacy, immunogenicity, and pharmacokinetic (PK) characteristics of SKG0106 in subjects with nAMD. Based on results from the phase 1 dose escalation study, the phase 2 expansion study will be conducted.

Official Title
A Multicenter, Open-label, Dose Escalation, Phase 1 Clinical Study and Randomized, Double-masked, Controlled, Dose Expansion Phase 2 Clinical Study to Evaluate the Safety, Preliminary Efficacy, Immunogenicity, and Pharmacokinetics of SKG0106 Intraocular Solution in Patients with Neovascular Age-Related Macular Degeneration (nAMD)

Conditions
Neovascular Age-Related Macular Degeneration

J. N. Weiss, *Clinical Trials in Age-Related Macular Degeneration Treatment*,
https://doi.org/10.1007/978-3-031-58803-7_4

Intervention/Treatment

- Genetic: SKG0106

Other Study ID Numbers

- SKG0106-101

Study Start (Estimated)
2023-10-30

Primary Completion (Estimated)
2025-11-30

Study Completion (Estimated)
2029-09-30

Enrollment (Estimated)
68

Study Type
Interventional

Phase
Phase 1 Phase 2

Study Contact
Name: Yongqin Wang
Phone Number: +86 18616737445
Email: yongqin.wang@skytx.com
United States
Texas Locations

Katy, Texas, United States, 77494
Retina Consultants of Texas

Contact
Marie Chin

Principal Investigator
Charles C Wykoff, MD

Virginia Locations

Norfolk, Virginia, United States, 23502
Wagner Kapoor Research Institute

Contact
Chris Riebling

Principal Investigator
Alan Wagner, MD

Eligibility Criteria
Description

Inclusion Criteria
- Voluntary and able to sign a dated ICF prior to any study-related procedures and able to complete the study as required by the protocol
- Aged ≥50 years at screening

Study Eye
- Diagnosis of nAMD as determined by the PI
- Active CNV lesions secondary to age-related macular degeneration (AMD)
- Subjects must have been responsive to anti-VEGF therapy as assessed by the PI prior to study treatment

Exclusion Criteria
- Any active intraocular or periocular infection or active intraocular inflammation (e.g., infectious conjunctivitis, keratitis, scleritis, endophthalmitis, infectious blepharitis, uveitis) in the study eye at baseline
- Retinal pigment epithelial tear in the study eye at screening
- Current vitreous hemorrhage in the study eye or history of vitreous hemorrhage within 4 weeks prior to baseline
- Any condition that, in the opinion of the investigator, may limit visual acuity improvement in the study eye
- History of retinal detachment or active retinal detachment in the study eye
- Any prior gene therapy

Ages Eligible for Study
50 Years and older (Adult, Older Adult)

Sexes Eligible for Study
All

Accepts Healthy Volunteers
No

Design Details
Primary Purpose: Treatment
Allocation: Nonrandomized
Interventional Model: Single Group Assignment
Masking: None (Open Label)

Arms and interventions

Participant group/arm	Intervention/treatment
Experimental: Phase I: Low dose SKG0106 One-Time Intraocular Injection Dose Level 1	Genetic: SKG0106 • SKG0106 is a recombinant adeno-associated virus (AAV) vector-based in vivo gene therapeutic product
Experimental: Phase I: Medium dose SKG0106 One-Time Intraocular Injection Dose Level 2	Genetic: SKG0106 • SKG0106 is a recombinant adeno-associated virus (AAV) vector-based in vivo gene therapeutic product

Experimental: Phase I: High dose SKG0106 One-Time Intraocular Injection Dose Level 3	Genetic: SKG0106 • SKG0106 is a recombinant adeno-associated virus (AAV) vector-based in vivo gene therapeutic product

Primary outcome measures

Outcome measure	Measure description	Time frame
Characteristics of dose-limiting toxicities (DLTs)		4 Weeks
Type, severity, and incidence of ocular and systemic adverse events (AEs)		52 Weeks

Secondary outcome measures

Outcome measure	Measure description	Time frame
Mean change from baseline in best corrected visual acuity (BCVA) at each visit	BCVA of the study eye is examined by the Early Treatment of Diabetic Retinopathy Study (ETDRS) testing at screening and baseline	52 Weeks
Mean change from baseline in central subfield thickness (CST) at each visit	Spectral domain optical coherence tomography (SD-OCT) will be performed to measure CST at screening and at each visit (prior to study drug injection, if available)	52 Weeks
Mean change from baseline in patient-reported outcome (VFQ-25) scale score at each visit	Both the total scale and subscale scores of the VFQ-25 is ranging from 0 to 100, and higher scores mean a better outcome	52 Weeks

Sponsor
Skyline Therapeutics (US) Inc.

Collaborators
No information provided

Investigators
No information provided

General Publications
No publications available

United States

Recruiting

4D-150 in Patients with Neovascular (Wet) Age-Related Macular Degeneration

ClinicalTrials.gov ID NCT05197270

Sponsor 4D Molecular Therapeutics
Information provided by 4D Molecular Therapeutics (Responsible Party)
Last Update Posted 2023-08-31

Study Overview

Brief Summary
Phase 1/2 dose-escalation and randomized, controlled, masked expansion trial in adults with wet AMD undergoing active anti-VEGF treatment

Detailed Description
This Phase 1/2 trial is a prospective, multicenter, Phase 1/2 dose-escalation and randomized, controlled, masked expansion trial in adults with wet AMD undergoing active anti-VEGF treatment who have demonstrated a clinical response consistent with anti-VEGF activity. The trial consists of Dose Escalation, Dose Expansion, Steroid Optimization, and Population Extension Cohorts.

After receiving one time administration of 4D-150 by intravitreal injection, subjects will undergo assessments at monthly intervals for 24 months to assess safety and efficacy outcomes. Only subjects who received 4D-150 will then enter a long-term follow-up (LTFU) period to assess long-term safety of 4D-150 gene therapy and duration of clinical activity through year 5 (60 months).

Official Title
A Phase 1/2 Dose-Escalation and Randomized, Controlled, Masked Expansion Trial of Intravitreal 4D-150 Gene Therapy in Adults with Neovascular (Wet) Age-Related Macular Degeneration

Conditions
Neovascular (Wet) Age-Related Macular Degeneration

Intervention/Treatment
- Biological: 4D-150 IVT
- Biological: Aflibercept IVT

Other Study ID Numbers
- 4D-150-C001
- Study Start (Actual)
- 2021-12-09

Primary Completion (Estimated)
2024-11

Study Completion (Estimated)
2025-11

Enrollment (Estimated)
150

Study Type
Interventional

Phase
Phase 1 and Phase 2

United States
Arizona Locations

Phoenix, Arizona, United States, 85016
Recruiting
Barnet Delaney Perkins Eye Center

Contact
Lori Slonecker
Lori.Slonecker@bdpec.com

Principal Investigator
Suhail Alam, M.D.

California Locations

Oxnard, California, United States, 93036
Recruiting
California Retina Consultants

Contact
Ellie Gonzalez
ellie@californiaretina.com

Principal Investigator
Dante Pieramici, M.D.

Sacramento, California, United States, 95841
Recruiting
Retinal Consultants Medical Group

Contact
Mira Cukrov
cukrovm@retinalmd.com

Principal Investigator
Joel Pearlman, M.D., Ph.D.

Colorado Locations

Lakewood, Colorado, United States, 80288
Recruiting
Colorado Retina Associates

Contact
Sara Shaw
sshaw@retinacolorado.com

Principal Investigator
Murtaza Adam, MD

Florida Locations

Deerfield Beach, Florida, United States, 33064
Recruiting
Rand Eye Institute

Contact
Damian Stega
dstega@randeye.com

Principal Investigator
Carl Danzig, MD

Gainesville, Florida, United States, 32607
Recruiting
Vitreo Retinal Associates

Contact
Jing Yang
jingzhang@vra-pa.com

Principal Investigator
Christine Kay, M.D.

Melbourne, Florida, United States, 32901
Recruiting
Florida Eye Associates

Contact
Yvonne Santiago
ysantiago@floridaeyeassociates.com

Principal Investigator
Vrinda Hershberger, M.D., Ph.D.

Pensacola, Florida, United States, 32503
Recruiting
Retinal Specialty Institute

Contact
Vera Watkins, R.N.
vwatkins@retinaspecialty.com

Principal Investigator
Sunil Gupta, M.D.

Tampa, Florida, United States, 33607
Recruiting
Retina Vitreous Associates of Florida

Contact
Allison Calvanese
acalvanese@rvaf.com

Principal Investigator
David Eichenbaum, M.D.

Illinois Locations

Oak Forest, Illinois, United States, 60452
Recruiting
University Retina and Macula Associates

Contact
Breanne Kirby
bkirby@uretina.com

Principal Investigator
Veeral Sheth, M.D.

Indiana Locations

Carmel, Indiana, United States, 46290
Recruiting
Retina Partners Midwest

Contact
Lorraine White
startup@midwesteye.com

Principal Investigator
Raj Maturi, MD

Maryland Locations

Hagerstown, Maryland, United States, 21740
Recruiting
Cumberland Valley Retina Consultants

Contact
Brittany Carson
BrittanyC@retinacare.net

Principal Investigator
Allen Hu, M.D.

Massachusetts Locations

Boston, Massachusetts, United States, 02114
Recruiting
Ophthalmic Consultants of Boston & Boston Eye Surgery and Laser Center

Contact
Sandy Chyong
schong@eyeboston.com

Principal Investigator
Jeffrey Heier, MD

Nevada Locations

Reno, Nevada, United States, 89502
Recruiting
Sierra Eye Associates

Contact
Naisha Shamim
nshamim@sierraeyeassociates.com

Principal Investigator
Arshad Khanani, M.D., M.A.

North Carolina Locations

Asheville, North Carolina, United States, 28803
Recruiting
Western Carolina Retinal Associates

Contact
McCayla Hall
mchall@aea1961.com

Principal Investigator
Cameron Stone, MD

Oregon Locations

Eugene, Oregon, United States, 97401
Recruiting
Verum Research, LLC

Contact
Ryan Lebien
rlebien@versumresearch.com

Principal Investigator
Albert Edwards, MD

Pennsylvania Locations

Bethlehem, Pennsylvania, United States, 18017
Recruiting
Mid Atlantic Retina

Contact
Ranya Girgis
dstega@randeye.com

Principal Investigator
Ajay Kuriyan, MD

South Carolina Locations

West Columbia, South Carolina, United States, 29169
Recruiting
Palmetto Retina Center, LLC

Contact
Pamala Tims
ptims@palmettoretina.com

Principal Investigator
John Wells, MD

Tennessee Locations

Nashville, Tennessee, United States, 37203
Recruiting
Tennessee Retina

Contact
Lisa Walden
LWalden@tnretina.com

Principal Investigator
Carl Awh, MD

Texas Locations

Austin, Texas, United States, 78705
Withdrawn
Austin Retina Associates

Austin, Texas, United States, 78750
Recruiting
Austin Clinical Research

Contact
Ivana Gunderson
igunderson@retinaresearchcenter.net

Principal Investigator
Fuad Makkouk, M.D.

Houston, Texas, United States, 77030
Recruiting
Retina Consultants of Texas

Contact
Chelsey Moore
chelsey.moore@retinaconsultantstexas.com

Principal Investigator
David Brown, M.D.

McAllen, Texas, United States, 78503
Recruiting
Valley Retina Institute, PA

Contact
Yesenia Salinas
yesenia.salinas@eyeptcare.com

Principal Investigator
Victor Gonzalez, M.D.

The Woodlands, Texas, United States, 77384
Recruiting
Retina Consultants of Texas

Contact
Kelly Reddin
kelly.reddin@retinaconsultantstexas.com

Principal Investigator
Charles Wykoff, M.D., Ph.D.

Washington Locations

Bellevue, Washington, United States, 98004
Recruiting
Pacific Northwest Retina LLC

Contact
Erdan Sun
e.sun@pnwretina.com

Principal Investigator
Todd Klesert, MD

Puerto Rico

Arecibo, Puerto Rico, 00612
Recruiting
Emanuelli Research and Development Center, LLC

Contact
Diane Perez
dperez@erdpr.com

Principal Investigator
Andres Emanuelli, MD

Eligibility Criteria
Description

Inclusion Criteria
- ≥50 years of age
- Diagnosed with macular CNV secondary to AMD
- BCVA ETDRS Snellen equivalent for dose escalation between ~20/32 and ~20/320, or for dose expansion and population extension between ~20/25 and ~20/200 for steroid optimization between ~20/25 and ~20/640
- Currently receiving anti-VEGF treatment in the study eye and has demonstrated a clinical response consistent with anti-VEGF activity within 12 months prior to screening

Exclusion Criteria
- Any condition preventing visual acuity improvement in the study eye
- Prior treatment with photodynamic therapy or retinal laser in the study eye
- History of uveitis in either eye
- Any other pre-existing eye conditions or surgical complications that would preclude participation in an interventional clinical trial or interfere with the interpretation of study endpoints

Ages Eligible for Study
50 Years and older (Adult, Older Adult)

Sexes Eligible for Study
All

Accepts Healthy Volunteers
No

Design Details
Primary Purpose: Treatment
Allocation: Randomized
Interventional Model: Sequential Assignment
Interventional Model Description: In Dose Escalation, the safety and tolerability of multiple dose levels of 4D-150 will be examined following an open-label, 3 + 3 dose

escalation design (n = 3–5 per dose level). In Dose Expansion, subjects (n = 50) will be randomized to receive one of 2 dose levels of 4D-150 (n = 20 for each dose level) based on results from Dose Escalation or aflibercept (n = 10). In Steroid Optimization (n = up to 40) and Population Extension (n = up to 45) Cohorts, subjects will be assigned sequentially to receive 4D-150 at doses cleared by the DSMC.

Masking: Single (Outcomes Assessor)

Masking Description: Dose Escalation will be open-label. During Dose Expansion, outcome assessors will be masked to treatment assignment. Other site personnel (including investigator) and subjects will be unmasked to treatment assignment but will be masked to 4D-150 dose level. The Sponsor and its representatives and the site dose preparer/pharmacist will be unmasked to treatment assignment. Steroid Optimization and Population Extension will be open-label

Arms and interventions

Participant group/arm	Intervention/treatment
Experimental: 4D-150 Dose Escalation up to 4 dose levels 4D-150 will be administered at the assigned dose level as a single dose IVT injection on Day 1	Biological: 4D-150 IVT • 4D-150: AAV-based gene therapy comprised of miRNA targeting VEGF-C and codon-optimized sequence encoding aflibercept
Experimental: 4D-150 Dose Expansion Dose 1 4D-150 will be administered at the assigned dose level as a single dose IVT injection on Day 1	Biological: 4D-150 IVT • 4D-150: AAV-based gene therapy comprised of miRNA targeting VEGF-C and codon-optimized sequence encoding aflibercept
Experimental: 4D-150 Dose Expansion Dose 2 4D-150 will be administered at the assigned dose level as a single-dose IVT injection on Day 1	Biological: 4D-150 IVT • 4D-150: AAV-based gene therapy comprised of miRNA targeting VEGF-C and codon-optimized sequence encoding aflibercept
Active Comparator: 4D-150 Dose Expansion Control Aflibercept at a fixed regimen will be administered	Biological: Aflibercept IVT • Commercially available Active Comparator Other Name: Eylea
Experimental: 4D-150 Steroid Optimization 4D-150 will be administered at the assigned dose level as a single-dose IVT injection on Day 1	Biological: 4D-150 IVT • 4D-150: AAV-based gene therapy comprised of miRNA targeting VEGF-C and codon-optimized sequence encoding aflibercept
Experimental: 4D-150 Population Extension Dose 1 4D-150 will be administered at the assigned dose level as a single-dose IVT injection on Day 1	Biological: 4D-150 IVT • 4D-150: AAV-based gene therapy comprised of miRNA targeting VEGF-C and codon-optimized sequence encoding aflibercept
Experimental: 4D-150 Population Extension Dose 2 4D-150 will be administered at the assigned dose level as a single-dose IVT injection on Day 1	Biological: 4D-150 IVT • 4D-150: AAV-based gene therapy comprised of miRNA targeting VEGF-C and codon-optimized sequence encoding aflibercept

Primary outcome measures

Outcome measure	Measure description	Time frame
Incidence and severity of treatment emergent adverse events (TEAEs) and serious adverse events (SAEs), including clinically significant changes in safety parameters		52 weeks

Secondary outcome measures

Outcome measure	Measure description	Time frame
Time to receiving the first supplemental aflibercept injection		52 weeks
Percentage of subjects requiring supplemental aflibercept injections over 52 weeks		52 weeks
Number of supplemental aflibercept injections over 52 weeks		52 weeks
Change from baseline in BCVA over time (up to 52 weeks) as assessed using the ETDRS Visual Acuity Chart		52 weeks
Change from baseline in central subfield thickness (CST) over time (up to 52 weeks) measured by spectral domain optical coherence tomography (SD-OCT)		52 weeks

Sponsor
4D Molecular Therapeutics

Collaborators
No information provided

Investigators
- Study Director: Chyong Nien, MD, 4D Molecular Therapeutics

General Publications
No publications available

United States

Recruiting

RGX-314 Gene Therapy Administered in the Suprachoroidal Space for Participants with Neovascular Age-Related Macular Degeneration (nAMD) (AAVIATE)

ClinicalTrials.gov ID NCT04514653

Sponsor AbbVie
Information provided by AbbVie (Responsible Party)
Last Update Posted 2023-05-22

Study Overview

Brief Summary

RGX-314 is being developed as a potential novel one-time gene therapy treatment for the treatment of neovascular (wet) age-related macular degeneration (wet AMD). Wet AMD is characterized by loss of vision due to new, leaky blood vessel formation in the retina. Wet AMD is a significant cause of vision loss in the United States, Europe, and Japan, with up to two million people living with wet AMD in these geographies alone. Current anti-VEGF therapies have significantly changed the landscape for the treatment of wet AMD becoming the standard of care due to their ability to prevent progression of vision loss in the majority of patients. These therapies, however, require life-long intraocular injections, typically repeated every 4–12 weeks in frequency, to maintain efficacy. Due to the burden of treatment, patients often experience a decline in vision with reduced frequency of treatment over time.

Detailed Description

This phase 2, randomized, dose-escalation study is designed to evaluate the efficacy, safety, and tolerability of RGX-314 gene therapy in subjects with nAMD. Approximately 115 participants who meet the inclusion/exclusion criteria will be enrolled into one of 6 cohorts. Participants will be randomized in Cohorts 1 and 2 to receive RGX-314 or ranibizumab control, and participants enrolled in Cohorts 3 through 5 will receive RGX-314. Participants enrolled in Cohort 6 will receive RGX-314 and will be randomized to one of two different post-procedural steroid regimens. Cohort 1 will evaluate RGX-314 Dose 1, Cohorts 2 and 3 will evaluate RGX-314 Dose 2, and Cohorts 4, 5, and 6 will evaluate RGX-314 Dose 3. Participants will be evaluated for efficacy, safety, and tolerability of RGX-314 throughout the study.

Official Title

A Phase 2, Randomized, Dose-escalation, Ranibizumab-controlled Study to Evaluate the Efficacy, Safety, and Tolerability of RGX-314 Gene Therapy Delivered Via One or Two Suprachoroidal Space (SCS) Injections in Participants with Neovascular Age-Related Macular Degeneration (nAMD) (AAVIATE)

Conditions

Neovascular Age-Related Macular Degeneration (nAMD)

Intervention/Treatment

- Genetic: RGX-314 Dose 1
- Genetic: RGX-314 Dose 2
- Biological: Ranibizumab
- Genetic: RGX-314 Dose 3
- Drug: Local steroid
- Drug: Topical steroid

Other Study ID Numbers

- RGX-314-2102
- Study Start (Actual)
- 2020-08-25

Primary Completion (Estimated)
2023-10

Study Completion (Estimated)
2024-01

Enrollment (Estimated)
115

Study Type
Interventional

Phase
Phase 2

Study Contact
Name: Patient Advocacy
Phone Number: 1-866-860-0117
Email: patientadvocacy@regenxbio.com
United States
Arizona Locations

Phoenix, Arizona, United States, 85014
Recruiting
Phoenix Location

Contact
Principal Investigator

California Locations

Bakersfield, California, United States, 93309
Active, not recruiting
Bakersfield Location

Beverly Hills, California, United States, 90211
Recruiting
Beverly Hills Location

Contact
Principal Investigator

Mountain View, California, United States, 94040
Recruiting
Mountain View Location

Contact
Principal Investigator

Poway, California, United States, 92064
Recruiting
Poway Location

Contact
Principal Investigator

Santa Barbara, California, United States, 93103
Active, not recruiting
Santa Barbara Location

Georgia Locations

Augusta, Georgia, United States, 30909
Recruiting
Augusta Location

Contact
Principal Investigator

Maryland Locations

Baltimore, Maryland, United States, 21287
Recruiting
Baltimore Location

Contact
Principal Investigator

Massachusetts Locations

Boston, Massachusetts, United States, 02114
Recruiting
Boston Location

Contact
Principal Investigator

Nevada Locations

Reno, Nevada, United States, 89502
Recruiting
Reno Location

Contact
Principal Investigator

New Mexico Locations

Albuquerque, New Mexico, United States, 87109
Recruiting
Albuquerque Location

Contact
Principal Investigator

Pennsylvania Locations

Philadelphia, Pennsylvania, United States, 19107
Recruiting
Philadelphia Location

Contact
Principal Investigator

Tennessee Locations

Germantown, Tennessee, United States, 38138
Active, not recruiting
Germantown Location

Nashville, Tennessee, United States, 37203
Active, not recruiting
Nashville Location

Texas Locations

The Woodlands, Texas, United States, 77384
Active, not recruiting
Woodlands Location

Eligibility Criteria
Description

Inclusion Criteria

- Age >/= 50 and </= 89
- Diagnosis of CNV secondary to age-related macular degeneration in the study eye
- Participants must have demonstrated a meaningful response to anti-VEGF therapy
- Willing and able to provide written, signed informed consent for this study

Exclusion Criteria

- CNV or macular edema in the study eye secondary to any causes other than AMD
- Subfoveal fibrosis or atrophy in study eye
- Participants who have had a prior vitrectomy
- Active or history of retinal detachment in the study eye
- History of intravitreal therapy in the study eye, such as intravitreal steroid injection or investigational product (IP), other than anti-VEGF therapy, in the 6 months prior to study entry
- Received any gene therapy
- Any condition preventing visualization of the fundus or VA improvement in the study eye, e.g., cataract
- History of intraocular surgery in the study eye within 12 weeks of study entry
- Receipt of any IP within 30 days of study entry or 5 half-lives of the IP
- Myocardial infarction, cerebrovascular accident, or transient ischemic attacks within 6 months of study entry
- Cohorts 1–5 only: Uncontrolled glaucoma in the study eye
- COHORT 6 ONLY:

- Active or history of glaucoma or ocular hypertension in the study eye
- Certain OCT characteristics including: Large Pigment Epithelial Detachments (PED) and clinically significant Epiretinal Membrane (ERM) in the study eye at Visit 1

Note: Other inclusion/exclusion criteria apply.

Ages Eligible for Study
50 Years to 89 Years (Adult, Older Adult)

Sexes Eligible for Study
All

Accepts Healthy Volunteers
No

Design Details
Primary Purpose: Treatment
Allocation: Randomized
Interventional Model: Sequential Assignment
Masking: Single (Outcomes Assessor)
Masking Description: The vision examiners and central reading center (CRC) graders will be masked, meaning they will be unaware of the participants' treatment assignment. All other individuals affiliated with the study (investigators, all study center personnel apart from the vision examiners, the participants, all Sponsor staff, all staff affiliated with the contract research organization, and all CRC staff apart from the CRC graders) will have knowledge of the treatment assignment

Arms and interventions

Participant group/arm	Intervention/treatment
Active Comparator: Ranibizumab control Control treatment arm	Biological: Ranibizumab • Ranibizumab (anti-VEGF agent)
Experimental: RGX-314 Treatment Arm (Dose 1) RGX-314 Dose 1	Genetic: RGX-314 Dose 1 • AAV8 vector containing a transgene for anti-VEGF fab (Dose 1) • Other Names: –Combination Product
Experimental: RGX-314 Treatment Arm (Dose 2) RGX-314 Dose 2	Genetic: RGX-314 Dose 2 • AAV8 vector containing a transgene for anti-VEGF fab (Dose 2) • Other Names: –Combination Product
Experimental: RGX-314 Treatment Arm (Dose 3) RGX-314 Dose 3	Genetic: RGX-314 Dose 3 • AAV8 vector containing a transgene for anti-VEGF fab (Dose 3) • Other Names: –Combination Product

Experimental: RGX-314 Treatment Arm (Dose 3) and Local Steroid RGX-314 Dose 3 and Local Steroid	Genetic: RGX-314 Dose 3 • AAV8 vector containing a transgene for anti-VEGF fab (Dose 3) • Other Names: –Combination Product Drug: Local steroid • Local Steroid
Experimental: RGX-314 Treatment Arm (Dose 3) and Topical Steroid RGX-314 Dose 3 and Topical Steroid	Genetic: RGX-314 Dose 3 • AAV8 vector containing a transgene for anti-VEGF fab (Dose 3) • Other Names: –Combination Product Drug: Topical steroid • Topical steroid

Primary outcome measures

Outcome measure	Measure Description	Time frame
To evaluate the mean change in Best Corrected Visual Acuity (BCVA) for RGX-314 compared with ranibizumab monthly	The scale used is the early treatment diabetic retinopathy study (ETDRS) letter score from 0 to 100 and higher score being better vision	40 weeks

Secondary outcome measures

Outcome measure	Measure description	Time frame
Evaluate the safety and tolerability of RGX-314	Incidence of overall and ocular adverse events (AEs) and serious adverse events (SAEs)	52 weeks
Evaluate the incidence of ocular inflammation following the administration of RGX-314	Proportion of participants who experience ocular inflammation following SCS RGX-314 administration	52 weeks
Evaluate the effect of RGX-314 on choroidal neovascularization (CNV) lesion growth and leakage	Mean change from baseline in CNV lesion size and leakage area based on fluorescein angiography (FA) at Week 52	52 weeks
Evaluate the effect of RGX-314 on BCVA	Mean change from baseline in BCVA to Week 52	52 weeks
Evaluate the effect of RGX-314 on central retinal thickness (CRT)	Mean change from baseline in CRT as measured by spectral domain-optical coherence tomography (SD-OCT) to Week 40 and Week 52	52 weeks
Assess the need for supplemental anti-vascular endothelial growth factor (VEGF) therapy in participants who receive RGX-314 treatment	Mean supplemental anti-VEGF injection annualized rate in the RGX-314 treatment arm through Week 40 and Week 52	52 weeks
Evaluate the concentration of RGX-314 transgene product (TP) in aqueous humor and serum	Mean change from baseline and Week 54 in serum RGX-314 TP concentration over time	52 weeks

Sponsor
AbbVie

Collaborators
No information provided

Investigators
No information provided

General Publications
No publications available

United States

Recruiting

Safety and Efficacy of ADVM-022 in Treatment-Experienced Patients with Neovascular Age-Related Macular Degeneration [LUNA]

ClinicalTrials.gov ID NCT05536973

Sponsor Adverum Biotechnologies, Inc.
Information provided by Adverum Biotechnologies, Inc. (Responsible Party)
Last Update Posted 2023-05-26

Study Overview

Brief Summary
Neovascular or wet age-related macular degeneration (nAMD) is a degenerative ocular disease associated with the infiltration of abnormal blood vessels in the retina from the underlying choroid layer and is a leading cause of blindness in patients over 65 years of age. The abnormal angiogenic process in nAMD is stimulated and modulated by vascular endothelial growth factor (VEGF). Treatment of nAMD requires frequent intravitreal (IVT) injections of VEGF inhibitors (anti-VEGF) administered every 4–16 weeks. ADVM-022 (AAV.7m8-aflibercept) is a gene therapy product being developed for the treatment of nAMD and offers the potential for sustained intraocular expression of aflibercept following a single IVT injection. ADVM-022 is designed to reduce the current treatment burden which often results in undertreatment and vision loss in patients with nAMD receiving anti-VEGF therapy in clinical practice.

Detailed Description
This Phase 2, multi-center, randomized, double-masked, parallel group study is designed to evaluate the safety, tolerability, and efficacy of a single IVT injection of ADVM-022 at one of two doses (2 × 10^11 vg/eye [2E11] or 6 × 10^10 vg/eye [6E10]) accompanied by one of four prophylactic corticosteroid treatment regimens.

Up to 72 anti-VEGF treatment-experienced study participants meeting the eligibility criteria will be randomized between the 2E11 vg/eye and 6E10 vg/eye ADVM-022 doses each with 4 prophylaxis arms for a total of 8 treatment arms, and only one eye per study participant will be selected as the study eye.

Safety, tolerability, and efficacy will be evaluated for a period of approximately 1 year from baseline.

Official Title
A Multi-Center, Randomized, Double-Masked Phase 2 Study to Assess Safety and Efficacy of ADVM-022 (AAV.7m8-aflibercept) in Anti-VEGF Treatment-Experienced Patients with Neovascular (Wet) Age-Related Macular Degeneration (nAMD) [LUNA]

Conditions
Neovascular Age-Related Macular Degeneration

Intervention/Treatment
- Genetic: ADVM-022
- Genetic: ADVM-022

Other Study ID Numbers
- ADVM-022-11
- Study Start (Actual)
- 2022-08-23

Primary Completion (Estimated)
2024-02

Study Completion (Estimated)
2024-02

Enrollment (Estimated)
72

Study Type
Interventional

Phase
Phase 2

Study Contact
Name: Sharri Adams-Edwards
Phone Number: (650) 649-1373
Email: LUNA-Clinops@adverum.com

Study Contact Backup
Name: Adam Turpcu, PhD
Phone Number: (650) 649-1012
Email: aturpcu@adverum.com

United States
Arizona Locations

Phoenix, Arizona, United States, 85020
Recruiting
Adverum Clinical Site 178

Phoenix, Arizona, United States, 85053
Recruiting
Adverum Clinical Site 126

Tucson, Arizona, United States, 85704
Recruiting
Adverum Clinical Site 159

California Locations

Beverly Hills, California, United States, 90211
Recruiting
Adverum Clinical Site 100

Encino, California, United States, 91436
Recruiting
Adverum Clinical Site 172

Fullerton, California, United States, 92835
Recruiting
Adverum Clinical Site 169

Pasadena, California, United States, 91105
Recruiting
Adverum Clinical Site 170

Poway, California, United States, 92064
Recruiting
Adverum Clinical Site 174

Riverside, California, United States, 92505
Recruiting
Adverum Clinical Site 164

Sacramento, California, United States, 95817
Recruiting
Adverum Clinical Site 166

Santa Barbara, California, United States, 93103
Recruiting
Adverum Clinical Site 175

Colorado Locations

Lakewood, Colorado, United States, 80228
Recruiting
Adverum Clinical Site 116

Connecticut Locations

Waterford, Connecticut, United States, 06385
Recruiting
Adverum Clinical Site 165

Florida Locations

Deerfield Beach, Florida, United States, 33064
Recruiting
Adverum Clinical Site 124

Fort Lauderdale, Florida, United States, 33308
Recruiting
Adverum Clinical Site 176

Jacksonville, Florida, United States, 32216
Recruiting
Adverum Clinical Site 168

Hawaii Locations

'Aiea, Hawaii, United States, 96701
Recruiting
Adverum Clinical Site 149

Michigan Locations

Detroit, Michigan, United States, 48201
Recruiting
Adverum Clinical Site 167

Royal Oak, Michigan, United States, 48073
Recruiting
Adverum Clinical Site 161

Mississippi Locations

Southaven, Mississippi, United States, 38671
Recruiting
Adverum Clinical Site 163

Nebraska Locations

Omaha, Nebraska, United States, 68105
Recruiting
Adverum Clinical Site 177

Nevada Locations

Reno, Nevada, United States, 89502
Recruiting
Adverum Clinical Site 119

New Jersey Locations

Cherry Hill, New Jersey, United States, 08034
Recruiting
Adverum Clinical Site 146

Teaneck, New Jersey, United States, 07666
Recruiting
Adverum Clinical Site 171

South Carolina Locations

West Columbia, South Carolina, United States, 29169
Recruiting
Adverum Clinical Site 122

South Dakota Locations

Rapid City, South Dakota, United States, 57701
Recruiting
Adverum Clinical Site 144

Tennessee Locations

Nashville, Tennessee, United States, 37203
Recruiting
Adverum Clinical Site 101

Texas Locations

Abilene, Texas, United States, 79606
Recruiting
Adverum Clinical Site 123

Austin, Texas, United States, 78705
Recruiting
Adverum Clinical Site 154

Bellaire, Texas, United States, 77401
Recruiting
Adverum Clinical Site 108

McAllen, Texas, United States, 78503
Recruiting
Adverum Clinical Site 162

San Antonio, Texas, United States, 78240
Recruiting
Adverum Clinical Site 151

The Woodlands, Texas, United States, 77384
Recruiting
Adverum Clinical Site 107

West Virginia Locations

Morgantown, West Virginia, United States, 26506
Not yet recruiting
Adverum Clinical Site 152

France
Loire-Atlantique Locations

Nantes, Loire-Atlantique, France, 44093
Not yet recruiting
Adverum Clinical Site 502

Rhône Locations

Lyon, Rhône, France, 69004
Not yet recruiting
Adverum Clinical Site 501

Val-de-Marne Locations

Créteil, Val-de-Marne, France, 94000
Not yet recruiting
Adverum Clinical Site 500

United Kingdom

London, United Kingdom, EC1V 2PD
Not yet recruiting
Adverum Clinical Site 600

Oxford, United Kingdom, OX3 9DU
Not yet recruiting
Adverum Clinical Site 601

Eligibility Criteria
Description

Inclusion Criteria
- Male or female participants, ≥ 50 years of age
- Willing and able to provide written, signed informed consent for this study
- Demonstrated a meaningful response to anti-VEGF therapy
- Participants must be under active anti-VEGF treatment for wet AMD and received a minimum of 2 injections within 4 months prior to screening for the treatment of choroidal neovascularization secondary to nAMD in the study eye
- BCVA ETDRS Snellen equivalent between ≤20/25 and ≥20/320

Exclusion Criteria

- Any condition that could affect the interpretation of results or render the participant at high risk of treatment complications in the opinion of the Investigator
- Ocular or periocular infection or intraocular inflammation in either eye within 1 month prior to or at the Randomization Visit (Day -7)
- Uncontrolled diabetes or HbA1c ≥ 7.0%
- History or evidence of significant uncontrolled concomitant disease within 6 months of the Screening visit
- Any history of ongoing bleeding disorders or INR >3.0
- History or evidence of macular or retinal disease other than nAMD
- History or evidence of retinal detachment or retinal pigment epithelium rip/tear
- Uncontrolled ocular hypertension or glaucoma
- Prior treatment with photodynamic therapy or retinal laser for the treatment of nAMD
- Any history of vitrectomy or any other vitreoretinal surgery within 3 months prior to the Randomization Visit (Day -7)
- Prior treatment with gene therapy at any time or any nongene therapy investigational treatment or medical device in the study eye within 3 months of the Screening Visit or 5 half-lives of the investigational medicinal product

Ages Eligible for Study

50 Years and older (Adult, Older Adult)

Sexes Eligible for Study

All

Accepts Healthy Volunteers

No

Design Details

Primary Purpose: Treatment
Allocation: Randomized
Interventional Model: Parallel Assignment
Masking: Double (Participant Investigator)

Arms and interventions

Participant group/arm	Intervention/treatment
Experimental: Dose 1 A single intravitreal injection of ADVM-022 2E11 vg/eye	Genetic: ADVM-022 • A single IVT injection of 2E11 vg/eye ADVM-022 dose in combination with one (1) of four (4) corticosteroid treatment regimens
Experimental: Dose 2 A single intravitreal injection of ADVM-022 6E10 vg/eye	Genetic: ADVM-022 • A single IVT injection of 6E10 vg/eye ADVM-022 dose in combination with one (1) of four (4) corticosteroid treatment regimens

Primary outcome measures

Outcome measure	Measure description	Time frame
Severity of ocular and nonocular adverse events	Incidence of ocular and nonocular adverse events	From Baseline to Week 52
Incidence of ocular and nonocular adverse events	Incidence of ocular and nonocular adverse events	From Baseline to Week 52
Mean change in best corrected visual acuity (BCVA) from Baseline	BCVA measured by Early Treatment Diabetic Retinopathy Study (ETDRS)	Week 52

Secondary outcome measures

Outcome measure	Measure description	Time frame
Percentage of participants from Baseline who lose/gain at least 5, 10, or 15 letters in Best Corrected Visual Acuity (BCVA)	BCVA measured by ETDRS	Week 52
Mean change in BCVA from Baseline	BCVA measured by ETDRS	Week 26
Percentage of participants who are supplemental aflibercept injection-free	Supplemental anti-VEGF treatments required post therapy	Week 52
Percentage reduction in anti-VEGF injections	Supplemental anti-VEGF treatments required post therapy to the year prior	Week 52
Mean change in Central Subfield Thickness (CST) from Baseline	To evaluate the effect of ADVM-022 on CST	Week 52
Percentage of participants without CST fluctuations > 50 μm	To evaluate the effect of ADVM-022 on CST	Week 52
Mean number of CST fluctuations > 50 μm from Baseline	To evaluate the effect of ADVM-022 on CST	Week 52

Sponsor
Adverum Biotechnologies, Inc.

Collaborators
- Parexel

Investigators
- Study Director: Adam Turpcu, PhD, Adverum Biotechnologies, Inc.

General Publications
No publications available

United States

Recruiting

A Study of EXG102-031 in Patients with wAMD (Everest)

ClinicalTrials.gov ID NCT05903794

Sponsor Exegenesis Bio
Information provided by Exegenesis Bio (Responsible Party)
Last Update Posted 2023-07-27

Study Overview

Brief Summary
In neovascular (wet) age-related macular degeneration (nAMD), the macula, or the part of the eye that provides the clear, detailed central vision, is being affected by abnormal blood vessel growth and leakage. This leakage affects the vision over time and can lead to severe blurriness or blinding. EXG102-031 was made to block the extra vessel formation which would lead to less leakage affecting the vision. Before EXG102-031 can be tested for its efficacy (if it makes vision better), it must be tested to see if it is safely tolerated to confirm it can continue to be studied in more patients with nAMD.

Detailed Description
Age-related macular degeneration (AMD) is a major cause of blindness and visual impairment in older adults. The wet form of AMD, also called neovascular AMD (nAMD), usually causes faster vision loss than the dry form. The most common current treatments of nAMD are products that inhibit vascular endothelial growth factor (VEGF) (including ranibizumab (LUCENTIS®, Genentech) and aflibercept (EYLEA®, Regeneron) and are delivered by intravitreal injections at 4–16 week intervals and continued indefinitely. This Phase I, open-label, multiple-cohort, dose-escalation study is designed to evaluate the safety and tolerability of EXG102-031 gene therapy in subjects with previously treated nAMD. Safety will be assessed over 52 weeks after the administration of EXG102-031, and study participants will be followed for a total of five years after they receive the investigational administration of EXG102-031.

Official Title
An Open-label, Dose-escalation Study to Evaluate the Safety and Tolerability of Gene Therapy with EXG102-031 in Participants with Neovascular Age-Related Macular Degeneration

Conditions
Neovascular (Wet) Age-related Macular Degeneration (nAMD)

Intervention/Treatment
- Biological: EXG102-031

Other Study ID Numbers
- EXG102-031 (211)
- Study Start (Actual)
- 2023-07-24

Primary Completion (Estimated)
2024-12-31

Study Completion (Estimated)
2025-12-31

Enrollment (Estimated)
6

Study Type
Interventional

Phase
Phase 1

Study Contact
Name: Anna Oughton, PharmD
Phone Number: 12153536621
Email: quality-exg102-031@exegenesisbio.com
United States
Pennsylvania Locations

Erie, Pennsylvania, United States, 16507
Recruiting
Erie Retina Research

Contact
Bethany Bielak-Scott
814-456-4241 ext 5408 b.scott.research@pm.me

Eligibility Criteria
Description

Inclusion Criteria
- Male or female, age ≥ 50 years of age
- Diagnosis of nAMD and current active lesion in the study eye at Screening
- An ETDRS BCVA letter scores between 73 and 19 letters in the study eye
- Response to anti-VEGF treatment during Screening
- The study eye must be a pseudophakic lens (post-cataract surgery status)
- Voluntarily agree to participate in the clinical trial, understand the trial procedures, and be capable of signing the informed consent form before screening

Exclusion Criteria
- Presence of any ocular disease or history of disease in the study eye other than nAMD that may affect central visual acuity and/or macular detection, including

retinal detachment, or in the opinion of the investigator could limit VA improvement in the study eye
- Presence in the study eye of CNV or macular edema due to causes other than AMD
- Presence in the study eye of scarring, fibrosis, or atrophy involving the macula
- Subretinal hemorrhage accumulating in the center of the macula of the test eye, with an area of hemorrhage ≥4 optic disc diameters
- Active ocular infection in either eye
- Presence of advanced glaucoma or uncontrolled glaucoma in the study eye
- History of intraocular surgery in the study eye within 90 days of screening
- Prior receipt of any ocular or systemic gene therapy agent

Ages Eligible for Study
50 Years and older (Adult, Older Adult)

Sexes Eligible for Study
All

Accepts Healthy Volunteers
No

Design Details
Primary Purpose: Treatment
Allocation: N/A
Interventional Model: Sequential Assignment
Interventional Model Description: Dose-escalation Study with two cohorts of three participants in each.
Masking: None (Open Label)

Arms and interventions

Participant group/arm	Intervention/treatment
Experimental: EXG102-031 Each participant will receive a single subretinal injection of EXG102-031 in the study eye. Participants will be enrolled into one of two dosage groups sequentially, and the dose administered will be determined based on which study group the participant is enrolled in	Biological: EXG102-031 • EXG102-031 is a recombinant adeno-associated virus (rAAV) expressing an angiopoietin domain and VEGF receptor (ABD-VEGFR) fusion protein. EXG102-031 will be administered by subretinal injection into one eye of each participant

Primary outcome measures

Outcome measure	Measure description	Time frame
Evaluation of safety and tolerability	Frequency, type, and intensity of ocular and nonocular adverse events (AEs) and serious adverse events (SAEs)	Throughout 52 weeks

Secondary outcome measures

Outcome measure	Measure description	Time frame
Evaluation of potential efficacy	Change from baseline in best corrected visual acuity (BCVA) measured by the ETDRS method	52 weeks post administration
Evaluation of potential safety	Frequency, type, and intensity of ocular and nonocular adverse events (AEs) and serious adverse events (SAEs)	Through week 24
Evaluation of supplementary therapy injections received	Average number of doses of anti-vascular endothelial growth factor (VEGF) supplemental therapy received	Throughout 52 weeks post administration

Sponsor
Exegenesis Bio

Collaborators
No information provided

Investigators
- Principal Investigator: Arshad Khanani, MD, Sierra Eye Associates

General Publications
No publications available

United States

Recruiting

Pivotal 2 Study of RGX-314 Gene Therapy in Participants with nAMD (ASCENT)

ClinicalTrials.gov ID NCT05407636

Sponsor AbbVie
Information provided by AbbVie (Responsible Party)
Last Update Posted 2023-08-21

Study Overview

Brief Summary
RGX-314 is being developed as a novel one-time gene therapy for the treatment of neovascular (wet) age-related macular degeneration (wet AMD). Wet AMD is characterized by loss of vision due to new, leaky blood vessel formation in the retina. Wet AMD is a significant cause of vision loss in the United States, Europe, and Japan, with up to two million people living with wet AMD in these geographies alone. Current anti-VEGF therapies have significantly changed the landscape for

the treatment of wet AMD becoming the standard of care due to their ability to prevent progression of vision loss in the majority of patients. These therapies, however, require life-long intraocular injections, typically repeated every 4–4–12 weeks in frequency, to maintain efficacy. Due to the burden of treatment, patients often experience a decline in vision with reduced frequency of treatment over time. RGX-314 is being developed as a potential one-time treatment for wet AMD.

Detailed Description
This randomized, partially masked, controlled, Phase 3 clinical study will evaluate the efficacy and safety of RGX-314 gene therapy in participants with nAMD. The study will evaluate 2 dose levels of RGX-314 gene therapy relative to an active comparator. The primary endpoint of this study is mean change in best-corrected visual acuity (BCVA) of RGX-314 relative to aflibercept. Approximately 465 participants who meet the inclusion/exclusion criteria will be enrolled into one of 3 arms.

Official Title
A Randomized, Partially Masked, Controlled, Phase 3 Clinical Study to Evaluate the Efficacy and Safety of RGX-314 Gene Therapy in Participants with nAMD

Conditions
AMD
nAMD
Wet Age-Related Macular Degeneration
wAMD
WetAMD
CNV

Intervention/Treatment
- Genetic: RGX-314 Dose 1
- Genetic: RGX-314 Dose 2
- Biological: Aflibercept (EYLEA®)

Other Study ID Numbers
- RGX-314-3101
- Study Start (Actual)
- 2021-12-28

Primary Completion (Estimated)
2025-02

Study Completion (Estimated)
2025-12

Enrollment (Estimated)
465

Study Type
Interventional

Phase
Phase 3

Study Contact
Name: Patient Advocacy
Phone Number: +(1) 866-860-0117
Email: Patientadvocacy@regenxbio.com
United States
Arizona Locations

Mesa, Arizona, United States, 85016
Recruiting
Barnet Dulaney Perkins Eye Center

Phoenix, Arizona, United States, 85014
Recruiting
Retinal Consultants of Arizona

Phoenix, Arizona, United States, 85053
Recruiting
Retinal Research Institute

California Locations

Bakersfield, California, United States, 93309
Recruiting
California Retina Consultants

Beverly Hills, California, United States, 90211
Recruiting
Retina Vitreous Associates Medical Group

Campbell, California, United States, 95008
Recruiting
Retinal Diagnostic Center

Encino, California, United States, 91436
Recruiting
The Retina Partners

La Jolla, California, United States, 92093
Recruiting
UC San Diego

Poway, California, United States, 92064
Recruiting
Retina Consultants of San Diego

Sacramento, California, United States, 85841
Recruiting
Retinal Consultants Medical Group, Inc

Sacramento, California, United States, 95817
Recruiting
UC Davis

Santa Ana, California, United States, 92705
Recruiting
Orange County Retina Medical Group

Colorado Locations

Colorado Springs, Colorado, United States, 80909
Recruiting
Retina Consultants of Southern Colorado P.C.

Durango, Colorado, United States, 81303
Recruiting
Southwest Retina Consultants

Lakewood, Colorado, United States, 80228
Recruiting
Colorado Retina Associates

Longmont, Colorado, United States, 80503
Recruiting
Eye Care Center of Northern Colorado

Florida Locations

Fort Myers, Florida, United States, 33912
Recruiting
National Ophthalmic Research Institute

Gainesville, Florida, United States, 32607
Recruiting
Vitreo Retinal Associates PA

Lakeland, Florida, United States, 33805
Recruiting
Florida Retina Consultants

Orlando, Florida, United States, 32806
Recruiting
Florida Retina Institute

Pensacola, Florida, United States, 32503
Recruiting
Retina Specialty Institute

Pompano Beach, Florida, United States, 33064
Recruiting
Rand Eye Institute

Saint Petersburg, Florida, United States, 33711
Recruiting
Retina Vitreous Associates of Florida - Saint Petersburg

Winter Haven, Florida, United States, 33880
Recruiting
Center for Retina and Macular Disease

Georgia Locations

Marietta, Georgia, United States, 30060
Recruiting
Georgia Retina PC

Hawaii Locations

'Aiea, Hawaii, United States, 96701
Recruiting
Retina Consultants of Hawaii

Illinois Locations

Lemont, Illinois, United States, 60439
Recruiting
University Retina and Macula Associates, P.C.

Oak Forest, Illinois, United States, 60452
Recruiting
University Retina and Macula Associates, P.C.

Oak Park, Illinois, United States, 60304
Recruiting
Illinois Retina Associates

Springfield, Illinois, United States, 62702
Recruiting
Springfield Clinic

Indiana Locations

Indianapolis, Indiana, United States, 46290
Recruiting
MidWest Eye Institute

New Albany, Indiana, United States, 47150
Recruiting
John-Kenyon American Eye Institute

Iowa Locations

West Des Moines, Iowa, United States, 50266
Recruiting
Wolfe Eye Clinic

Maine Locations

Portland, Maine, United States, 04101
Recruiting
Maine Eye Center

Maryland Locations

Baltimore, Maryland, United States, 21204
Recruiting
Retina Specialists

Baltimore, Maryland, United States, 21287
Recruiting
Johns Hopkins University

Baltimore, Maryland, United States, 21287
Recruiting
Wilmer Eye Institute

Hagerstown, Maryland, United States, 21740
Recruiting
Mid Atlantic Reina Specialists

Massachusetts Locations

Boston, Massachusetts, United States, 02114
Recruiting
Massachusetts Eye and Ear Infirmary

Boston, Massachusetts, United States, 02114
Recruiting
Ophthalmic Consultants of Boston, Inc

Michigan Locations

Grand Blanc, Michigan, United States, 48439
Recruiting
Retina Associates of Michigan

Novi, Michigan, United States, 48375
Recruiting
Associated Retinal Consultants

Minnesota Locations

Edina, Minnesota, United States, 55435
Recruiting
Vitreo Retinal Surgery, PA

Nevada Locations

Reno, Nevada, United States, 89502
Recruiting
Sierra Eye Associates

New Jersey Locations

Bloomfield, New Jersey, United States, 07003
Recruiting
Envision Ocular, LLC

New York Locations

New York, New York, United States, 10032
Recruiting
Columbia University Irving Medical Center - Harness Eye Institute

Rochester, New York, United States, 14620
Recruiting
Retina Associates of Western New York

North Carolina Locations

Asheville, North Carolina, United States, 28803
Recruiting
Western Carolina Retina Associates P.A.

Durham, North Carolina, United States, 27705
Recruiting
Duke Eye Center

Hickory, North Carolina, United States, 28602
Recruiting
Greystone Eye

Ohio Locations
Cincinnati, Ohio, United States, 45242
Recruiting
Cincinnati Eye Institute

Cleveland, Ohio, United States, 44130
Recruiting
Retina Associates of Cleveland, Inc.

Cleveland, Ohio, United States, 44915
Recruiting
Cleveland Clinic

Columbus, Ohio, United States, 43212
Recruiting
The Ohio State University Eye & Ear Institute

Oklahoma Locations

Edmond, Oklahoma, United States, 73013
Recruiting
Retina Vitreous Center Research

Pennsylvania Locations

Philadelphia, Pennsylvania, United States, 19104
Recruiting
Scheie Eye Institute

Philadelphia, Pennsylvania, United States, 19107
Recruiting
Mid Atlantic Retina

Pittsburgh, Pennsylvania, United States, 15213
Recruiting
University of Pittsburgh Medical Center

South Carolina Locations

Beaufort, South Carolina, United States, 29902
Recruiting
Retina Consultants of Charleston

Charleston, South Carolina, United States, 29414
Recruiting
Retina Consultants of Charleston

Florence, South Carolina, United States, 29501
Recruiting
Palmetto Retina Center LLC

Ladson, South Carolina, United States, 29456
Recruiting
Retina Consultants of Charleston

Tennessee Locations

Chattanooga, Tennessee, United States, 37421
Recruiting
Southeastern Retina Associates

Germantown, Tennessee, United States, 38138
Recruiting
Charles Retina Institute

Johnson City, Tennessee, United States, 37604
Recruiting
Southeastern Retina Associates

Nashville, Tennessee, United States, 37203
Recruiting
Tennessee Retina Center Murfreesboro

Nashville, Tennessee, United States, 37232
Recruiting
Vanderbilt University Medical Center

Texas Locations

Abilene, Texas, United States, 79606-1224
Recruiting
Retina Research Institute of Texas

Abilene, Texas, United States, 79606
Recruiting
West Texas Retina Consultants - Abilene

Arlington, Texas, United States, 76012
Recruiting
Texas Retina Associates

Austin, Texas, United States, 78705
Recruiting
Retina Consultants of Austin

Austin, Texas, United States, 78750
Recruiting
Austin Clinical Research, LLC

Bellaire, Texas, United States, 77401
Recruiting
Retina Consultants of Texas

Burleson, Texas, United States, 76028
Recruiting
Star Retina

Dallas, Texas, United States, 75231
Recruiting
Ophthalmology Surgery Center of Dallas

Dallas, Texas, United States, 75231
Recruiting
Texas Retina Associates

Round Rock, Texas, United States, 78681
Recruiting
Austin Retina Associates

San Antonio, Texas, United States, 78240
Recruiting
Retina Associates of South Texas, P.A.

San Antonio, Texas, United States, 78240
Recruiting
Retina Consultants of Texas

San Antonio, Texas, United States, 78251
Recruiting
Brown Retina Institute

Southlake, Texas, United States, 76092
Recruiting
Retina Center of Texas - Southlake

Utah Locations

Salt Lake City, Utah, United States, 84107
Recruiting
Rocky Mountain Retina Consultants

Virginia Locations

Lynchburg, Virginia, United States, 24502
Recruiting
Piedmont Eye Center

Norfolk, Virginia, United States, 23502
Recruiting
Wagner Macula & Retina Center

Richmond, Virginia, United States, 23235
Recruiting
Retina Institute of Virginia

Washington Locations

Bellevue, Washington, United States, 98004
Recruiting
Pacific Northwest Retina

Bellevue, Washington, United States, 98004
Recruiting
Vitreoretinal Associates of Washington

Silverdale, Washington, United States, 98383
Recruiting
Retina Center Northwest

Spokane, Washington, United States, 99204
Recruiting
Spokane Eye Clinical Research

Canada

Québec, Canada, G1S 4L8
Recruiting
CHU de Quebec-Universite Laval

Alberta Locations

Calgary, Alberta, Canada, T2H 0C8
Recruiting
Calgary Retina Consultants

Edmonton, Alberta, Canada, T5H 0X5
Recruiting
Alberta Retina Research Corporation

Ontario Locations

Ottawa, Ontario, Canada, K2B 7E9
Recruiting
Retina Centre of Ottawa

Puerto Rico

Arecibo, Puerto Rico, 00612
Recruiting
Emanuelli Research and Development Center

Eligibility Criteria
Description

Inclusion Criteria
- Age $\geq$ 50 years and $\leq$ 89 years
- An ETDRS BCVA letter score between $\leq$78 and $\geq$40 in the study eye
- Diagnosis of subfoveal CNV secondary to AMD in the study eye previously treated with anti-VEGF
- Must be pseudophakic (at least 12 weeks postcataract surgery) in the study eye
- Willing and able to provide written, signed informed consent for this study
- Participants must have demonstrated a meaningful response to anti-VEGF therapy at study entry

Exclusion Criteria
- CNV or macular edema in the study eye secondary to any causes other than AMD
- Subfoveal fibrosis or atrophy in the study eye
- Any condition in the investigator's opinion that could limit VA improvement in the study eye
- Active or history of retinal detachment or current retinal tear in the study eye
- Advanced glaucoma or history of secondary glaucoma in the study eye
- Myocardial infarction, cerebrovascular accident, or transient ischemic attack within the past 6 months.

- History of intraocular surgery in the study eye within 12 weeks prior to Screening Visit 1
- History of intravitreal therapy in the study eye, such as intravitreal steroid injection or investigational product, other than anti-VEGF therapy, in the 6 months prior to Screening Visit 1.
- Prior treatment with gene therapy

Ages Eligible for Study
50 Years to 89 Years (Adult, Older Adult)

Sexes Eligible for Study
All

Accepts Healthy Volunteers
No

Design Details
Primary Purpose: Treatment
Allocation: Randomized
Interventional Model: Parallel Assignment
Interventional Model Description: 2 RGX-314 treatment arms, 1 control arm (aflibercept)
Masking: Single (Participant)
Masking Description: Care Provider, Investigator, Outcomes Assessor

Arms and interventions

Participant group/arm	Intervention/treatment
Experimental: RGX-314 Dose 1 RGX-314 Dose 1 administered via subretinal delivery one time	Genetic: RGX-314 Dose 1 • AAV8 vector containing a transgene for anti-VEGF Fab (Dose 1)
Experimental: RGX-314 Dose 2 RGX-314 Dose 2 administered via subretinal delivery one time	Genetic: RGX-314 Dose 2 • AAV8 vector containing a transgene for anti-VEGF Fab (Dose 2)
Active Comparator: Control Arm Aflibercept administered via intravitreal injection approximately every 8 weeks	Biological: Aflibercept (EYLEA®) • 2.0 mg (0.05 mLsolution) administered by intravitreal injection approximately every 8 weeks after 3 monthly injections Other Names: • Eylea (anti-VEGF agent)

Primary outcome measures

Outcome measure	Measure description	Time frame
Mean change from baseline in Best Corrected Visual Acuity (BCVA)	BCVA measured by Early Treatment Diabetic Retinopathy Study (ETDRS)	At Week 54

Secondary outcome measures

Outcome measure	Measure description	Time frame
Incidences of ocular and overall Serious Adverse Events (SAEs)	Incidences of ocular and overall Serious Adverse Events	At Week 54
Mean change from baseline in BCVA	BCVA measured by ETDRS	At Week 54 (RGX-314 randomized participants only)
Mean change from baseline in CRT and CPT as measured by SD-OCT	CRT and CPT as measured by SD-OCT	At Week 54 and Week 90
Mean reduction in supplemental anti-VEGF injection annualized rate compared with the prior year of therapy	Supplemental anti-VEGF treatments required post therapy to the year prior	Through Week 54 and Week 108
Mean supplemental anti-VEGF injection annualized rate in the RGX-314 arms	Supplemental anti-VEGF treatments required post therapy to the year prior	Through Week 54 and Week 108
Aqueous RGX-314 TP concentrations	Observation of concentration of RGX-314 in the aqueous humor over time	At Week 14, Week 38, Week 54, Week 74, Week 90 and Week 108

Sponsor
AbbVie

Collaborators
No information provided

Investigators
No information provided

General Publications
No publications available

United States

Recruiting

Pivotal 1 Study of RGX-314 Gene Therapy in Participants with nAMD (ATMOSPHERE)

ClinicalTrials.gov ID NCT04704921

Sponsor AbbVie
Information provided by AbbVie (Responsible Party)
Last Update Posted 2023-05-22

Study Overview

Brief Summary

RGX-314 is being developed as a novel one-time gene therapy for the treatment of neovascular (wet) age-related macular degeneration (wet AMD). Wet AMD is characterized by loss of vision due to new, leaky blood vessel formation in the retina. Wet AMD is a significant cause of vision loss in the United States, Europe, and Japan, with up to two million people living with wet AMD in these geographies alone. Current anti-VEGF therapies have significantly changed the landscape for treatment of wet AMD becoming the standard of care due to their ability to prevent progression of vision loss in the majority of patients. These therapies, however, require life-long intraocular injections, typically repeated every 44–12 weeks in frequency, to maintain efficacy. Due to the burden of treatment, patients often experience a decline in vision with reduced frequency of treatment over time. RGX-314 is being developed as a potential one-time treatment for wet AMD.

Detailed Description

This randomized, partially masked, controlled, Phase 2b/3 clinical study will evaluate the efficacy and safety of RGX-314 gene therapy in participants with nAMD. The study will evaluate 2 dose levels of RGX-314 relative to an active comparator. The primary endpoint of this study is the mean change in best-corrected visual acuity (BCVA) of RGX-314 relative to ranibizumab. Approximately 300 participants who meet the inclusion/exclusion criteria will be enrolled into one of three arms.

Official Title

A Randomized, Partially Masked, Controlled, Phase 2b/3 Clinical Study to Evaluate the Efficacy and Safety of RGX-314 Gene Therapy in Participants with nAMD (ATMOSPHERE)

Conditions

AMD
nAMD
Wet Age-Related Macular Degeneration
wAMD
Wet AMD
CNV

Intervention/Treatment

- Genetic: RGX-314
- Genetic: RGX-314
- Biological: Ranibizumab (LUCENTIS®)

Other Study ID Numbers

- RGX-314-2104
- Study Start (Actual)
- 2020-12-29

Primary Completion (Estimated)
2025-05

Study Completion (Estimated)
2026-05

Enrollment (Estimated)
300

Study Type
Interventional

Phase
Phase 2 Phase 3

Study Contact
Name: Patient Advocacy
Phone Number: 1-866-860-0117
Email: patientadvocacy@regenxbio.com
United States
Arizona Locations

Phoenix, Arizona, United States, 85014
Recruiting
Retinal Consultants of Arizona, Ltd.

Sun City, Arizona, United States, 85351
Recruiting
Barnet Dulaney Perkins Eye Center—Phoenix

California Locations

Beverly Hills, California, United States, 90211
Recruiting
Retina-Vitreous Associates Medical Group

Campbell, California, United States, 95008
Recruiting
Retinal Diagnostic Center

Encino, California, United States, 91436
Recruiting
The Retina Partners—Encino

Fullerton, California, United States, 92835
Recruiting
Retina Consultants of Orange County—Fullerton Office

Irvine, California, United States, 92697
Recruiting
University of California Irvine—School of Medicine—The Gavin Herbert Eye Institute

Los Angeles, California, United States, 90033
Recruiting
Doheny Eye Institute - Doheny Eye Center—Arcadia

Mountain View, California, United States, 94040
Recruiting
Northern California Retina Vitreous Associates Medical Group, Inc. —Mountain View Office

Pasadena, California, United States, 91107
Recruiting
California Eye Specialists Medical Group Inc.—Pasadena

Poway, California, United States, 92064
Recruiting
Retina Consultants San Diego

Sacramento, California, United States, 95819
Recruiting
Retina Consultants

San Francisco, California, United States, 94109
Recruiting
West Coast Retina Medical Group—San Francisco Office

Contact
San Francisco 1 Location

San Francisco, California, United States, 94143
Recruiting
UCSF Medical Center—Retina and Vitreous Clinic

Santa Ana, California, United States, 92705
Recruiting
Orange County Retina Medical Group

Santa Barbara, California, United States, 85014
Recruiting
California Retina Consultants

Colorado Locations

Colorado Springs, Colorado, United States, 80909
Recruiting
Retina Consultants of Southern Colorado PC—Colorado Springs

Durango, Colorado, United States, 81301
Recruiting
Southwest Retina Consultants

Lakewood, Colorado, United States, 80401
Recruiting
Colorado Retina Associates (CRA)—Red Rocks Medical Center Location

Connecticut Locations

Waterford, Connecticut, United States, 06385
Recruiting
Retina Group of New England—New London

Florida Locations

Gainesville, Florida, United States, 32607
Recruiting
Vitreo Retinal Associates PA—The Millennium Center

Lakeland, Florida, United States, 33805-2908
Not yet recruiting
Florida Retina Consultants—Lakeland

Miami, Florida, United States, 33136
Recruiting
Bascom Palmer Eye Institute—University of Miami Health System

Pensacola, Florida, United States, 32503
Recruiting
Retina Specialty Institute—Pensacola

Saint Petersburg, Florida, United States, 33711
Recruiting
Retina Vitreous Associates of Florida (RVA)—Saint Petersburg

Tallahassee, Florida, United States, 32308
Not yet recruiting
Southern Vitreoretinal Associates, P.L.

Georgia Locations

Augusta, Georgia, United States, 30909
Active, not recruiting
Southeast Retina Center

Marietta, Georgia, United States, 30060
Recruiting
Georgia Retina PC—Marietta

Hawaii Locations

Aiea, Hawaii, United States, 96701
Recruiting
Retina Consultants of Hawaii (RCH) —Pali Momi Medical Center Location

Illinois Locations

Chicago, Illinois, United States, 60612
Recruiting
Illinois Eye and Ear Infirmary at UI Health UIC

Lemont, Illinois, United States, 60439
Recruiting
University Retina and Macula Associates, P.C.—Lemont Office

Oak Forest, Illinois, United States, 60452
Recruiting
University Retina and Macula Associates, PC—Oak Forest

Springfield, Illinois, United States, 62702
Not yet recruiting
Springfield Clinic

Springfield, Illinois, United States, 62703
Not yet recruiting
Springfield Clinic

Indiana Locations

Indianapolis, Indiana, United States, 46290
Recruiting
Midwest Eye Institute

New Albany, Indiana, United States, 47150
Recruiting
John-Kenyon American Eye Institute—New Albany

Kansas Locations

Shawnee Mission, Kansas, United States, 66204
Recruiting
Retina Associates, P.A.—Shawnee Mission

Maryland Locations

Baltimore, Maryland, United States, 21209
Recruiting
The Retina Care Center, LLC

Baltimore, Maryland, United States, 21287
Recruiting
The Johns Hopkins Hospital—Wilmer Eye Institute—East Baltimore

Hagerstown, Maryland, United States, 21740
Recruiting
Cumberland Valley Retina Consultants (CVRC)

Massachusetts Locations

Boston, Massachusetts, United States, 02114
Recruiting
Ophthalmic Consultants of Boston, Inc.

Michigan Locations

Grand Blanc, Michigan, United States, 48439-8301
Not yet recruiting
Retina Associates of Michigan—Grand Blanc Office

Royal Oak, Michigan, United States, 48073
Recruiting
Associated Retinal Consultants P.C.

Minnesota Locations

Minneapolis, Minnesota, United States, 55435
Recruiting
VitreoRetinal Surgery, PA—Edina Location

Contact
Location

Rochester, Minnesota, United States, 55905
Recruiting
Mayo Clinic—Minnesota

Nevada Locations

Reno, Nevada, United States, 89502
Recruiting
Sierra Eye Associates

New Mexico Locations

Albuquerque, New Mexico, United States, 87109
Recruiting
Eye Associates of New Mexico—Albuquerque—Retina Center Location

New York Locations

Great Neck, New York, United States, 11021
Recruiting
Long Island Vitreoretinal Consultants—Great Neck

North Carolina Locations

Durham, North Carolina, United States, 27705
Recruiting
Duke Eye Center—Erwin Road—Duke University Medical Center

Winston-Salem, North Carolina, United States, 27157
Not yet recruiting
Wake Forest Baptist Medical Center

Ohio Locations

Cincinnati, Ohio, United States, 45242
Recruiting
Cincinnati Eye Institute—Blue Ash

Cleveland, Ohio, United States, 44130
Recruiting
Retina Associates of Cleveland, Inc.—Middleburg Heights Office

Cleveland, Ohio, United States, 44195
Recruiting
Cleveland Clinic

Oklahoma Locations

Edmond, Oklahoma, United States, 73013
Recruiting
Retina Vitreous Center (RVC)

Oregon Locations

Portland, Oregon, United States, 97221
Recruiting
Retina Northwest, PC

Pennsylvania Locations

Erie, Pennsylvania, United States, 16507-1429
Recruiting
Erie Retinal Surgery, Inc

Philadelphia, Pennsylvania, United States, 19107
Recruiting
Mid Atlantic Retina—Philadelphia

South Carolina Locations

Ladson, South Carolina, United States, 29456-4118
Recruiting
Charleston Neuroscience Institute

South Dakota Locations

Rapid City, South Dakota, United States, 57701
Recruiting
Black Hills Regional Eye Institute

Tennessee Locations

Germantown, Tennessee, United States, 38138
Recruiting
Charles Retina Institute

Texas Locations

Abilene, Texas, United States, 79606
Recruiting
West Texas Retina Consultants (WTRC)—Abilene Location

Austin, Texas, United States, 78705
Recruiting
Austin Retina Associates

Austin, Texas, United States, 78705
Recruiting
Retina Consultants of Austin

Austin, Texas, United States, 78750
Recruiting
Austin Clinical Research, LLC

Burleson, Texas, United States, 79606
Recruiting
Star Retina

Contact
Burleson Location

Dallas, Texas, United States, 75231
Recruiting
Texas Retina Associates

Fort Worth, Texas, United States, 76104
Not yet recruiting
Star Vision Consultants

San Antonio, Texas, United States, 78240-1657
Not yet recruiting
Retina Associates of South Texas, PA—San Antonio

San Antonio, Texas, United States, 78240-1657
Not yet recruiting
Retinal Consultants of San Antonio (RCSA)—Medical Center

Southlake, Texas, United States, 76092
Recruiting
Retina Center of Texas—Southlake

The Woodlands, Texas, United States, 77030
Recruiting
Retina Consultants of Texas—The Woodlands

Utah Locations

Salt Lake City, Utah, United States, 84107
Recruiting
Retina Associates of Utah, PC

Salt Lake City, Utah, United States, 84132
Recruiting
John A. Moran Eye Center—University of Utah Health Care

Virginia Locations

Virginia Beach, Virginia, United States, 23454
Recruiting
Wagner Macula & Retina Center

Washington Locations

Bellevue, Washington, United States, 98004-3779
Recruiting
Pacific Northwest Retina

Silverdale, Washington, United States, 98383-7849
Recruiting
Retina Center Northwest—Silverdale

Wisconsin Locations

Madison, Wisconsin, United States, 53705
Recruiting
University of Wisconsin Health—University Station Clinic

Eligibility Criteria
Description

Inclusion Criteria

- Age ≥50 years and ≤89 years
- An ETDRS BCVA letter score between ≤78 and ≥40 in the study eye
- Diagnosis of subfoveal CNV secondary to AMD in the study eye previously treated with anti-VEGF
- Must be pseudophakic (at least 12 weeks postcataract surgery) in the study eye
- Willing and able to provide written, signed informed consent for this study
- Participants must have demonstrated a meaningful response to anti-VEGF therapy at study entry

Exclusion Criteria

- CNV or macular edema in the study eye secondary to any causes other than AMD
- Subfoveal fibrosis or atrophy in the study eye
- Any condition in the investigator's opinion that could limit VA improvement in the study eye
- Active or history of retinal detachment in the study eye
- Uncontrolled glaucoma in the study eye
- History of intraocular surgery in the study eye within 12 weeks prior to Screening Visit 1
- History of intravitreal therapy in the study eye, such as intravitreal steroid injection or investigational product, other than anti-VEGF therapy, in the 6 months prior to Screening Visit 1
- Prior treatment with gene therapy
- Recent myocardial infarction, cerebrovascular accident, or transient ischemic attack within the past 6 months

Ages Eligible for Study
50 Years to 89 Years (Adult, Older Adult)

Sexes Eligible for Study
All

Accepts Healthy Volunteers
No

Design Details
Primary Purpose: Treatment
Allocation: Randomized
Interventional Model: Parallel Assignment
Interventional Model Description: 2 RGX-314 treatment arms, 1 control arm (ranibizumab)
Masking: Quadruple (Participant Care Provider Investigator Outcomes Assessor)
Masking Description: The administration of RGX-314 requires an outpatient surgical procedure performed in an operating room, while the active control, ranibizumab, is administered via intravitreal injection in an office setting. This study will be partially masked which will include masking of key study assessors and study drug dose

Arms and interventions

Participant group/arm	Intervention/treatment
Experimental: RGX-314 Dose 1 RGX-314 Dose 1 administered via subretinal delivery one time	Genetic: RGX-314 • AAV8 vector containing a transgene for anti-VEGF Fab (Dose 1)
Experimental: RGX-314 Dose 2 RGX-314 Dose 2 administered via subretinal delivery one time	Genetic: RGX-314 • AAV8 vector containing a transgene for anti-VEGF Fab (Dose 2)
Active Comparator: Control Arm Ranibizumab administered via intravitreal injection approximately every 28 days	Biological: Ranibizumab (LUCENTIS®) • 0.5 mg (0.05 mL of 10 mg/mL solution) was administered by intravitreal injection approximately every 28 days • Other Names: –Ranibizumab (anti-VEGF agent)

Primary outcome measures

Outcome measure	Measure description	Time frame
Mean change from baseline in Best Corrected Visual Acuity (BCVA)	BCVA measured by Early Treatment Diabetic Retinopathy Study (ETDRS)	At Week 54

Secondary outcome measures

Outcome measure	Measure description	Time frame
Incidences of ocular and overall adverse events (AEs)	Evaluate the safety and tolerability of RGX-314	Through Week 98
Mean change from baseline in BCVA	BCVA measured by ETDRS	At Week 98 (RGX-314 randomized participants only)
Mean change from baseline in Central Retinal Thickness (CRT) and Center Point Thickness (CPT) as measured by Spectral Domain Optical Coherence Tomography (SD-OCT)		At Week 54 and Week 98
Mean reduction in supplemental anti VEGF injection annualized rate compared with the prior 52 weeks preceding the first ranibizumab injection received as part of the Active Run-in Period (RGX 314 randomized participants)		Through Week 54 and Week 98
Mean supplemental anti-VEGF injection annualized rate in the RGX-314 arms		Through Week 54 and Week 98
Aqueous RGX-314 target protein (TP) concentrations		At Week 14, Week 26, Week 38, Week 54, and Week 98

Collaborators and Investigators

This is where you will find people and organizations involved with this study

Sponsor

AbbVie

Collaborators

No information provided

Investigators

No information provided

General Publications

No publications available

Canada

Recruiting

NG101 AAV Gene Therapy in Subjects with Wet Age-Related Macular Degeneration

ClinicalTrials.gov ID NCT05984927

Sponsor Neuracle Genetics, Inc
Information provided by Neuracle Genetics, Inc (Responsible Party)
Last Update Posted 2023-10-19

Study Overview

Brief Summary
This study will evaluate the safety, tolerability, and preliminary efficacy of NG101 AAV gene therapy administered by subretinal injections into a single selected eye as a single selected dose for patients with wet age-related macular degeneration (wAMD).

Detailed Description
This is a Phase 1/2a, multicenter, open-label, dose escalation study to evaluate the safety, tolerability, and preliminary efficacy of NG101 AAV gene therapy, administered by subretinal injection in patients with active wAMD symptoms. The study will be conducted at approximately 6 sites in Canada and the USA.

Official Title
A Phase 1/2a Open-label Study to Evaluate Safety, Tolerability, and Preliminary Efficacy of NG101 AAV Gene Therapy in Subjects with Wet Age-Related Macular Degeneration

Conditions
Age-Related Macular Degeneration

Intervention/Treatment
- Genetic: NG101 AAV gene therapy

Other Study ID Numbers
- NG101WA-01
- Study Start (Actual)
- 2023-09-08

Primary Completion (Estimated)
2025-01

Study Completion (Estimated)
2030-01

Enrollment (Estimated)
18

Study Type
Interventional

Phase
Phase 1 Phase 2

Study Contact
Name: Sheila Yi
Phone Number: 770-296-7301
Email: wetamd@neuraclegen.com

Study Contact Backup
Name: Hea Reung Park
Email: wetamd@neuraclegen.com
Canada
Ontario Locations

Toronto, Ontario, Canada, M8X 2X3
Recruiting
Vitreous Retina Macula Specialists of Toronto

Contact
Tatjana Sukovic
tatjana@vrmto.com

Eligibility Criteria
Description

Inclusion Criteria
- Subjects ≥50 and ≤89 years of age with a diagnosis of active subfoveal CNV secondary to wAMD in the Study Eye
- BCVA between 20/63 and 20/400 in the Study Eye, with BCVA decrement primarily attributable to wAMD
- Administration of at least 3 anti-VEGF injections in the past 6 months, the most recent of which was within 2 months prior to Screening.
- Must be pseudophakic (status post cataract surgery) in the Study Eye
- Female subjects must be either: (1) of nonchildbearing potential; or (2) of childbearing potential and using an acceptable method of birth control with a negative pregnancy test
- Willing and able to provide written, signed informed consent after the nature of the study has been explained and prior to the performance of any study-related procedures
- Willingness and ability to comply with the schedule for follow-up visits and postoperative evaluations

Exclusion Criteria

- CNV or macular edema in the Study Eye secondary to any causes other than AMD
- Any condition preventing visual acuity improvement in the Study Eye, e.g., fibrosis, atrophy, or retinal pigment epithelial tear in the center of the macula
- Any ophthalmic condition that precludes adequate ophthalmic examination or requires ancillary testing
- Retinal detachment or history of retinal detachment in the Study Eye
- Active uncontrolled glaucoma with intraocular pressure (IOP) $\geq$ 30 mmHg despite treatment with more than 2 glaucoma medications, advanced glaucoma with cup-to-disc ratio of $\geq$0.9, visual field defects secondary to glaucoma that involve the macula, and/or optic atrophy from glaucoma
- History of intravitreal therapy in the Study Eye, such as intravitreal steroid injection or an investigational product, other than anti-VEGF therapy, in the 6 months prior to Screening
- History of vitrectomy, trabeculectomy, glaucoma tube-shunt procedure, minimally invasive glaucoma surgery (MIGS) device, or other filtration surgery in the Study Eye
- Any prior treatment with photodynamic therapy or retinal laser for the treatment of wAMD
- Any prior therapeutic radiation in the region of the Study Eye such as whole brain radiation, proton beam radiation, gamma knife treatment, or plaque brachytherapy
- Any previous intraocular or refractive surgery on the Study Eye within 6 months
- Any previous gene therapy in the Study Eye
- Presence of an ocular implant in the Study Eye at Screening, excluding intraocular lens and custom flex iris prosthesis
- Any diabetic retinopathy or other retinal vascular disease including retinal vein occlusion, retinal artery occlusion, retinal arterial macro aneurysm, ocular ischemic syndrome, retinal vasculitis, vitritis, and posterior uveitis
- Any medically uncontrolled diabetes, defined as HbA1C > 8.0
- History of ocular melanoma
- History of any known inherited retinal disease
- Currently taking any anticoagulant therapy, which is deemed medically necessary and cannot be permanently stopped at least 2 weeks prior to NG101 injection, excluding prophylactic low-dose aspirin therapy
- Any underlying systemic diseases such as severe cardiovascular, cerebrovascular, and neurodegenerative diseases, including active malignancy and immunocompromised conditions
- Active hepatitis B or C
- History of human immunodeficiency virus (HIV), active tuberculosis, and/or syphilis
- Any significant illness that would preclude study compliance and follow-up
- Subjects who, in the Investigator's opinion, lack the mental capacity to provide written informed consent for study participation

Ages Eligible for Study
50 Years to 89 Years (Adult, Older Adult)

Sexes Eligible for Study
All

Accepts Healthy Volunteers
No

Design Details
Primary Purpose: Treatment
Allocation: Nonrandomized
Interventional Model: Sequential Assignment
Interventional Model Description: Dose Escalation Study with 3 dose cohorts
Masking: None (Open Label)

Arms and interventions

Participant group/arm	Intervention/treatment
Experimental: NG101 Gene Therapy Group 1 Single subretinal injection of $1x10^9$ vector genomes of NG101 AAV gene therapy	Genetic: NG101 AAV gene therapy • Subretinal injection of NG101 (a nonreplicating adeno-associated virus serotype 8 (AAV8) vector • Other Names: –NG101
Experimental: NG101 Gene Therapy Group 2 Single subretinal injection of $3x10^9$ vector genomes of NG101 AAV gene therapy	Genetic: NG101 AAV gene therapy • Subretinal injection of NG101 (a nonreplicating adeno-associated virus serotype 8 (AAV8) vector • Other Names: –NG101
Experimental: NG101 Gene Therapy Group 3 Single subretinal injection of $8x10^9$ vector genomes of NG101 AAV gene therapy	Genetic: NG101 AAV gene therapy • Subretinal injection of NG101 (a nonreplicating adeno-associated virus serotype 8 (AAV8) vector • Other Names: –NG101

Primary outcome measures

Outcome measure	Measure description	Time frame
Adverse Events	Incidence and severity of ocular and nonocular adverse events (AEs) for each cohort	Day 0 (pre-treatment) and Week 24

Secondary outcome measures

Outcome measure	Measure description	Time frame
Ocular and Nonocular Adverse Events after week 24	Incidence and severity of ocular and nonocular AEs after Week 24 to Week 260 for each cohort	Day 0 (pre-treatment) and from Week 24 to Week 260
Systemic Immunogenic Response	Change in concentration of expressed aflibercept protein in vitreous samples	Day 0, week 12, week 24, week 52, and week 104

Systemic Immunogenic Response	Change in concentration of expressed aflibercept protein in serum samples	Day -7 week 4, week 12, and week 104
Systemic Immunogenic Response	Change in AAV vector (NG101) genome copies as measured by PCR in blood samples	Day -7, week 4, and week 12
Systemic Immunogenic Response	Change in concentration of Anti-NG101 Transgene protein antibodies, Anti-AAV8 Neutralizing antibodies, and Anti-AAV8 Antibodies in serum samples	Day -7, Week 4, week 8, week 12, week 24, week 52, and week 104
Signs of CNV Activity	Change of 1 or more signs of CNV activity assessed by optical coherence tomography	At every visit from Screening through Week 104
Central Retinal Thickness (CRT)	Change in CRT assessed with OCT	from Screening to Weeks 260
Best Corrected Visual Acuity (BCVA)	Change in BCVA assessed with Early Treatment Diabetic Retinopathy Study (ETDRS) scale	from Screening to Week 260
Cumulative Number of Rescue Therapy Injections	The cumulative number of rescue therapy injections per subject to maintain CNV control	From Week 24 to Week 260

Sponsor
Neuracle Genetics, Inc

Collaborators
- ORA, Inc.

Investigators
- Principal Investigator: Christopher D Riemann, MD, Neuracle Genetics, Inc. Medical Director

General Publications
No publications available

China

Recruiting

Safety and Tolerability of KH631 Gene Therapy in Participants with Neovascular Age-Related Macular Degeneration

ClinicalTrials.gov ID NCT05657301

Sponsor Chengdu Origen Biotechnology Co., Ltd.
Information provided by Chengdu Kanghong Pharmaceutical Group Co., Ltd. (Chengdu Origen Biotechnology Co., Ltd.) (Responsible Party)
Last Update Posted 2023-08-23

Study Overview

Brief Summary
VAN-2201 is Phase I clinical trial to assess the safety and tolerability of KH631 in subjects with neovascular AMD. KH631 is gene therapy designed to deliver a protein which targets and blocks VEGF via an adeno-associated viral vector. The standard of care for patients with neovascular AMD are anti-VEGF treatments, which have demonstrated improvement in vision and reduction in fluid. A one-time placement of a product which inhibits VEGF has the potential to reduce the patient burden of regular intraocular injections.

Detailed Description
The VAN-2201 clinical trial is a multicenter, open-label, dose-escalating clinical study. The primary objective of the study will be to establish a safe and tolerable dose range in subjects with neovascular AMD. Five dose cohorts are planned to be included in the study, with approximately five subjects per cohort. Subjects who meet the eligibility criteria (i.e., all the inclusion and no exclusion criteria) will be enrolled to receive KH631. KH631 will be delivered at the dose level according to the cohort via intraocular injection. Subjects will be seen monthly until the primary outcome measurement at 24 weeks and through week 52. The subjects will be continued to followed with regular visits until they complete the 104 week visit.

Official Title
A Phase I, Open-label, Multicenter, Dose-Escalating Study to Evaluate the Safety and Tolerability of KH631 Gene Therapy in Participants with Neovascular Age-Related Macular Degeneration

Conditions
Age-Related Macular Degeneration

Intervention/Treatment
- Drug: KH631

Other Study ID Numbers
- VAN-2201

Study Start (Estimated)
2023-08

Primary Completion (Estimated)
2026-09

Study Completion (Estimated)
2027-09

Enrollment (Estimated)
25

Study Type
Interventional

Phase
Phase 1

Study Contact
Name: Sponsor Clinical Contact
Phone Number: +1 267-644-6708
Email: van2201@cnkh.com
United States
Texas Locations

Katy, Texas, United States, 77494
Recruiting
Kanghong Investigative Site

Eligibility Criteria
Description

Inclusion Criteria

- Males and Females ages 50–85 (inclusive) with a study eye which meets the following criteria:
  - Previously received IVT treatment of anti-VEGF for neovascular AMD, with documented response to anti-VEGF therapy during the first 2 weeks of screening b. active macular CNV lesion secondary to AMD evidenced by SD-OCT c. Have a ETDRS BCVA letter score of 63 to 19 (approximately 20/63 to 20/400 Snellen equivalent) in the study eye at Screening for the first subject in each cohort (sentinel subject), followed by ETDRS BCVA letter score of 73 to 19 (approximately 20/40 to 20/400 Snellen equivalent) for the rest of the subjects each cohort; d. Pseudophakia in the study eye, with ocular media to permit high-quality fundus imaging at screening and allow planned vitrectomy and subretinal injection; e. Are willing and able to sign the study written informed consent form (ICF).

Exclusion Criteria

- Have had any prior ocular or systemic treatment (investigational or approved) or surgery for the treatment of neovascular AMD except IVT anti-VEGF
- Retinal pigment epithelial tears or rips at screening
- Any history or the presence of vitreous hemorrhage
- Have any condition preventing visual acuity improvement
- Have any other cause of CNV; prior pars plana vitrectomy or scleral buckling or retinal detachment surgery; macular hole, Epiretinal membrane or vitreo-macular traction; full thickness macular hole
- History of intraocular or periocular surgery in the prior 3 months
- Prior trabeculectomy or other filtration surgery
- Any use of long-acting intraocular steroids, including implants, within six months prior

Ages Eligible for Study
50 Years to 85 Years (Adult, Older Adult)

Sexes Eligible for Study
All

Accepts Healthy Volunteers

No

Design Details

Primary Purpose: Treatment
Allocation: N/A
Interventional Model: Single Group Assignment
Masking: None (Open Label)

Arms and interventions

Participant group/arm	Intervention/treatment
Experimental: KH631 Dose 1 KH631 One-Time Intraocular Injection Dose Level 1	Drug: KH631 • KH631: AAV vector containing a coding sequence for an anti-VEGF protein
Experimental: KH631 Dose 2 KH631 One-Time Intraocular Injection Dose Level 2	Drug: KH631 • KH631: AAV vector containing a coding sequence for an anti-VEGF protein
Experimental: KH631 Dose 3 KH631 One-Time Intraocular Injection Dose Level 3	Drug: KH631 • KH631: AAV vector containing a coding sequence for an anti-VEGF protein
Experimental: KH631 Dose 4 KH631 One-Time Intraocular Injection Dose Level 4	Drug: KH631 • KH631: AAV vector containing a coding sequence for an anti-VEGF protein
Experimental: KH631 Dose 5 KH631 One-Time Intraocular Injection Dose Level 5	Drug: KH631 • KH631: AAV vector containing a coding sequence for an anti-VEGF protein

Primary outcome measures

Outcome measure	Measure description	Time frame
Safety (Type, Severity, and Incidence of ocular and systemic AEs and SAEs)	Type, severity, and incidence of ocular and systemic AEs and SAEs	52 Weeks
Best Corrected Visual Acuity	Change in Best Corrected Visual Acuity	52 Weeks

Secondary outcome measures

Outcome measure	Measure description	Time frame
Safety (type, severity, and incidence of ocular and systemic AEs and SAEs)	Type, severity, and incidence of ocular and systemic AEs and SAEs	104 Weeks
Rescue Injections	Mean number of rescue injections	104 Weeks
Best Corrected Visual Acuity	Change in best corrected visual acuity	104 Weeks

Sponsor

Chengdu Origen Biotechnology Co., Ltd.

Collaborators

No information provided

Investigators
- Study Director: Avner Ingerman, MD, MSc, Vanotech Ltd.

General Publications
No publications available

China

Recruiting

Safety and Tolerability of KH631 Gene Therapy in Subjects with Neovascular Age-Related Macular Degeneration (nAMD)

ClinicalTrials.gov ID NCT05672121

Sponsor Chengdu Origen Biotechnology Co., Ltd.
Information provided by Chengdu Kanghong Pharmaceutical Group Co., Ltd. (Chengdu Origen Biotechnology Co., Ltd.) (Responsible Party)
Last Update Posted 2023-09-25

Study Overview

Brief Summary
KH631 is an adeno-associated virus (AAV) vector-based gene therapy for subretinal injection. The long-term, stable therapeutic protein after one time injection for nAMD could potentially reduce the treatment burden and maintain vision.

Official Title
A Phase I/II, Open-label, Multiple-cohort, Dose-Escalation Study to Evaluate the Safety and Tolerability of KH631 Gene Therapy in Subjects with Neovascular Age-related Macular Degeneration (nAMD)

Conditions
Age-Related Macular Degeneration

Intervention/Treatment
- Drug: KH631

Other Study ID Numbers
- KH631-40101
- Study Start (Actual)
- 2023-02-06

Primary Completion (Estimated)
2026-12-28

Study Completion (Estimated)
2026-12-28

Enrollment (Estimated)
42

Study Type
Interventional

Phase
Phase 1 Phase 2

Study Contact
Name: Qiang Zheng
Phone Number: 86 13880331037
Email: zhengqiang@cnkh.com

Study Contact Backup
Name: Ting Hu
Phone Number: 86 13880999215
Email: huting@cnkh.com
China

Beijing, China
Recruiting
Beijing Tongren Hospital, Capital Medical University

Contact
Wenbin Wei, PhD
86 13701255115 tr_weiwenbin@163.com

Eligibility Criteria
Description

Inclusion Criteria
- Are willing and able to sign the study written informed consent form (ICF)
- Men and women ≥50 and ≤85 years of age, diagnosed with nAMD at the Screening visit
- Subjects must be under active anti-VEGF treatment for nAMD and received a minimum of 3 injections within 6 months prior to screening
- Response to anti-VEGF therapy (response is defined as the reduction in CRT ≥ 50 μm or at least 30% reduction in the fluid by OCT compared to disease at the worst)
- BCVA between ≤20/63 and ≥20/400(≤63 and ≥19 Early Treatment Diabetic Retinopathy Study [ETDRS] letters) for the first patient in each cohort followed by BCVA between ≤20/40 and ≥20/400(≤73 and ≥19 ETDRS letters) for the rest of the cohort
- Must be pseudophakic (at least 3 months after intraocular lens implantation) in the study eye
- Female subjects must have been postmenopausal for at least 1 year

Exclusion Criteria

- Any other cause of CNV, including pathologic myopia, etc., or other diseases except nAMD influence the test of macular or affect the central visual acuity
- Presence of an implant, refractive media opacity affects fundus examination or narrow pupil of the study eye
- Active or history of retinal detachment in the study eye
- Uncontrolled glaucoma or ocular hypertension
- Have taken the drug known to have retinal toxicity
- History of intraocular surgery
- Uncontrolled hypertension despite medication at the screening visit

Ages Eligible for Study

50 Years to 85 Years (Adult, Older Adult)

Sexes Eligible for Study

All

Accepts Healthy Volunteers

No

Design Details

Primary Purpose: Treatment
Allocation: N/A
Interventional Model: Single Group Assignment
Masking: None (Open Label)

Arms and interventions

Participant group/arm	Intervention/treatment
Experimental: KH631 Dose 1 Dose 1: Administered by Subretinal injection. Dosage form: injection solution Dose: 200μL. Frequency of administration: one-time injection	Drug: KH631 • KH631: AAV vector containing a coding sequence for an anti-VEGF protein
Experimental: KH631 Dose 2 Dose 2: Administered by Subretinal injection. Dosage form: injection solution Dose: 200μL. Frequency of administration: one-time injection	Drug: KH631 • KH631: AAV vector containing a coding sequence for an anti-VEGF protein
Experimental: KH631 Dose 3 Dose 3: Administered by Subretinal injection. Dosage form: injection solution Dose: 200μL. Frequency of administration: one-time injection	Drug: KH631 • KH631: AAV vector containing a coding sequence for an anti-VEGF protein
Experimental: KH631 Dose 4 Dose 4: Administered by Subretinal injection. Dosage form: injection solution Dose: 200μL. Frequency of administration: one-time injection	Drug: KH631 • KH631: AAV vector containing a coding sequence for an anti-VEGF protein
Experimental: KH631 Dose 5 Dose 5: Administered by Subretinal injection. Dosage form: injection solution Dose: 200 μL. Frequency of administration: one-time injection	Drug: KH631 • KH631: AAV vector containing a coding sequence for an anti-VEGF protein

Primary outcome measures

Outcome measure	Measure description	Time frame
Safety	Incidence of AEs and SAEs	24 weeks
Change in best-corrected visual acuity	BCVA	52 weeks

Secondary outcome measures

Outcome measure	Measure description	Time frame
Safety	Incidence of AEs and SAEs	104 weeks
Change in best-corrected visual acuity	BCVA	104 weeks
Change in central retinal thickness	CRT	104 weeks
Change in area of retinal leakage	Leakage measured by FFA	104 weeks
Rescue injections	Mean number of rescue injections	104 weeks

Other outcome measures

Outcome measure	Measure description	Time frame
KH631 protein in aqueous fluid and blood	Exploratory	104 weeks
VEGF-A in aqueous fluid and blood	Exploratory	104 weeks

Sponsor
Chengdu Origen Biotechnology Co., Ltd.

Collaborators
No information provided

Investigators
- Principal Investigator: Wenbin Wei, PhD, Beijing Tongren Hospital Affiliated to Capital Medical University

General Publications
No publications available

China

Not Yet Recruiting

Gene Therapy for Wet AMD

ClinicalTrials.gov ID NCT05611424

Sponsor Frontera Therapeutics
Information provided by Frontera Therapeutics (Responsible Party)
Last Update Posted 2023-04-26

Study Overview

Brief Summary
FT-003 is a gene therapy product developed for the treatment of neovascular age-related macular degeneration (nAMD). Neovascular AMD is the main cause of blindness among elderly individuals. The available therapies for treating nAMD require life-long intravitreal (IVT) injections every 4–12 weeks to maintain efficacy. Administration of FT-003 has the potential to treat nAMD by providing durable expression of therapeutic levels of intraocular protein and maintaining the vision of patients. FT-003 is designed to reduce the current treatment burden which often results in undertreatment and vision loss in patients with nAMD receiving anti-VEGF therapy in clinical practice.

Official Title
An Open-label, Single-Center, Dose-Escalation Clinical Study to Evaluate the Safety, Tolerability, and Preliminary Efficacy of FT-003 in Subjects with Neovascular Age-Related Macular Degeneration

Conditions
Neovascular Age-Related Macular Degeneration

Intervention/Treatment
- Genetic: FT-003

Other Study ID Numbers
- FT003WA-1

Study Start (Estimated)
2023-05-01

Primary Completion (Estimated)
2024-11-30

Study Completion (Estimated)
2027-12-30

Enrollment (Estimated)
18

Study Type
Interventional

Phase
Phase 1

Study Contact
Name: Xinyan Li
Phone Number: +86-021-58206061
Email: Xinyan.li@fronteratherapeutics.com

Study Contact Backup
Name: Minghui Xue
Phone Number: +86-021-58206061
Email: minghui.xue@fronteratherapeutics.com
No location data

Eligibility Criteria
Description

Inclusion Criteria
- Subjects that are willing and able to follow study procedures
- Female or male patients ≥45 years old at the time of signing the ICF
- Clinically diagnosed with nAMD
- Presence of active CNV
- The best corrected visual acuity (BCVA) of the studied eye is ≤53 letters

Exclusion Criteria
- Presence of any other intraocular diseases other than nAMD in the studied eye that would affect the improvement of visual acuity and require treatment during the study for prevention or treatment of visual loss, as judged by the investigator.

Ages Eligible for Study
45 Years and older (Adult, Older Adult)

Sexes Eligible for Study
All

Accepts Healthy Volunteers
No

Design Details
Primary Purpose: Treatment
Allocation: Nonrandomized
Interventional Model: Single Group Assignment
Interventional Model Description: Neovascular Age-Related Macular Degeneration
Masking: None (Open Label)

Arms and interventions

Participant group/arm	Intervention/treatment
Experimental: FT003 Dose 1 Low dose of FT-003	Genetic: FT-003 • Administered via intraocular injection.
Experimental: FT003 Dose 2 Mid dose of FT-003	Genetic: FT-003 • Administered via intraocular injection.
Experimental: FT003 Dose 3 High dose of FT-003	Genetic: FT-003 • Administered via intraocular injection.

Primary outcome measures

Outcome measure	Measure description	Time frame
Safety and tolerability after FT-003 injection	Incidence and severity of AE (Common Terminology Criteria for Adverse Events 5.0)	At Week 52

Secondary outcome measures

Outcome measure	Measure description	Time frame
Changes in best-corrected visual acuity (BCVA) of the studied eye from baseline		At Week 52

Sponsor
Frontera Therapeutics

Collaborators
- The First Affiliated Hospital of Soochow University
- Tianjin Medical University Eye Hospital
- Peking Union Medical College Hospital
- The First Affiliated Hospital of Zhengzhou University

Investigators
- Principal Investigator: Peirong Lu, Professor, The First Affiliated Hospital of Soochou University
- Principal Investigator: Xiaorong Li, Professor, Tianjin Medical University Eye Hospital
- Principal Investigator: Hanyi Min, Peking Union Medical College Hospital
- Principal Investigator: Guangming Wan, The First Affiliated Hospital of Zhengzhou University

General Publications
No publications available

China

Recruiting

CRISPR/Cas13-Mediated RNA Targeting Therapy for the Treatment of nAMD Investigator-Initiated Trial (SIGHT-I)

ClinicalTrials.gov ID NCT06031727

Sponsor HuidaGene Therapeutics Co., Ltd.
Information provided by HuidaGene Therapeutics Co., Ltd. (Responsible Party)
Last Update Posted 2023-09-21

Study Overview

Brief Summary

Age-related macular degeneration (AMD) is a progressive disease leading to severe and irreversible vision loss of which the neovascular AMD (nAMD) accounted for 90% blindness in AMD. nAMD is primarily driven by the perturbation of vascular endothelial growth factor (VEGF). VEGF overexpression leads to abnormal growth of choroidal neovascularization (CNV), which is a hallmark of AMD. Although anti-VEGF agents are effective in treating nAMD, long-term efficacy decreases over time due to the need for repeated injections impacting patient compliance with the treatment regimen while patients still may lose vision during the 7th or 8th year of treatment. These frequent intravitreal injections can increase the risk of complications, including submacular hemorrhage, intraocular hypertension, inflammation, and retinal detachment. Furthermore, there are up to 46% of nAMD patients using anti-VEGF agents have shown poor response or have developed tachyphylaxis with anti-VEGF therapies. HG202 is a CRISPR/Cas13 RNA-editing therapy packaging novel high-fidelity Cas13 technology using one single AAV vector to partially knock down the expression of VEGFA and thus inhibit CNV formation in AMD patients who are either responsive or nonresponsive to anti-VEGF agents. The long-term, stable delivery of HG202 following a one (1) time gene-editing therapy treatment for nAMD could potentially reduce the frequent injection treatment burden of currently available therapies AND treat nAMD patients who are nonresponsive to anti-VEGF therapies and have no treatment.

Official Title

A Trial to Evaluate the Safety, Tolerability, and Efficacy of CRISPR-Cas13 RNA-editing Therapy Targeting Knockdown of Vascular Endothelial Growth Factor A (HG202) in the Treatment of Neovascular Age-Related Macular Degeneration (nAMD)

Conditions

Neovascular Age-Related Macular Degeneration (nAMD)

Intervention/Treatment

- Genetic: HG202

Other Study ID Numbers

- HG20201
- Study Start (Actual)
- 2023-09-04

Primary Completion (Estimated)

2024-12-31

Study Completion (Estimated)

2025-06-27

Enrollment (Estimated)

12

Study Type
Interventional

Phase
Early Phase 1

Study Contact
Name: Study Director
Phone Number: +86 021-25076143
Email: HG20201@huidagene.com
China
Shanghai Locations

Shanghai, Shanghai, China
Recruiting
Eye & ENT Hospital of Fudan University

Contact
Gezhi Xu, PhD
+86 18017316316 drxugezhi@163.com

Tianjing Locations

Tianjin, Tianjing, China
Recruiting
Tianjin Medical University Eye Hospital

Contact
Xiaorong Li, PhD
+86 18622818042 Xiaorli@163.com

Eligibility Criteria
Description

Inclusion Criteria
- Males or females ≥50 and ≤80 years at the time of signing the ICF
- Diagnosed with choroidal neovascularization (CNV) secondary to AMD in the study eye
- Best-corrected visual acuity (BCVA) ranged from 73 to 23 early treatment diabetic retinopathy study (ETDRS) letter score (corresponding to 20/32 to 20/320 of Snellen visual acuity) in the study eye
- BCVA in the nonstudy eye had an ETDRS letter score of 19 (equivalent to Snellen visual acuity20/400) and above
- Able to perform visual acuity and retinal function tests and able and willing to comply with study procedures for this clinical trial

Responsive Subjects
- History of need for and responsive to anti-VEGF therapy in the study eye

Nonresponsive Subjects

- History of receiving anti-VEGF therapy but is resistant to treatment, which is defined as a. complete or near-complete remission of subretinal fluid after the initial 3 doses of anti-VEGF agents and then no improvement (less than 50μm reduction) or deterioration of CRT by OCT

Exclusion Criteria

- Subretinal hemorrhage, scarring, or fibrosis of greater than 50% of the total lesion in the study eye
- Any condition in the Investigator's opinion that could limit visual improvement in the study eye
- Other ocular diseases that may affect central vision in the study eye (e.g., retinal vein occlusion, retinal detachment, macular hole, optic nerve disease, etc.)
- Presence of CNV not due to nAMD in the study eye
- Uncontrolled glaucoma in the study eye
- Active intraocular inflammation or a history of uveitis in either eye
- History or the presence of corneal dystrophy in the study eye
- Subjects with immunodeficiency diseases prone to opportunistic infections
- History of other intraocular surgery in the study eye within 3 months prior to the baseline that in the Investigator's opinion could impact healing or study outcome interpretation
- Prior gene therapy or oligonucleotide therapy
- History of acute coronary syndrome, myocardial infarction, coronary revascularization, cerebrovascular accident, or transient ischemic attack within 6 months prior to the Screening Visit
- Other conditions judged by the investigator as inappropriate for the study

Ages Eligible for Study
50 Years to 80 Years (Adult, Older Adult)

Sexes Eligible for Study
All

Accepts Healthy Volunteers
No

Design Details
Primary Purpose: Treatment
Allocation: N/A
Interventional Model: Single Group Assignment
Masking: None (Open Label)

Arms and interventions

Participant group/arm	Intervention/treatment
Experimental: HG202	Genetic: HG202 • Method of Administration: Once unilateral subretinal injection; the duration of the study is about 52 weeks for each subject including a 4 weeks screening period, enrollment/baseline visit, treatment visit, and 48 weeks follow-up period

Primary outcome measures

Outcome measure	Measure description	Time frame
Incidence and severity of ocular and systemic adverse events	Number of adverse events (AEs), serious adverse events (SAEs), and dose-limiting toxicities (DLTs)	24 weeks

Secondary outcome measures

Sponsor
HuidaGene Therapeutics Co., Ltd.

Collaborators
- Tianjin Medical University Eye Hospital
- Eye & ENT Hospital of Fudan University

Investigators
- Study Director: Study Director, Huidagene Therapeutics Co., Ltd.

Outcome measure	Measure description	Time frame
Incidence and severity of ocular and systemic adverse events	Number of adverse events (AEs), serious adverse events (SAEs), and dose-limiting toxicities (DLTs)	48 weeks
Change from baseline in best-corrected visual acuity (BCVA)	Change from baseline in BCVA as measured by Early Treatment Diabetic Retinopathy Study (ETDRS) chart in the study eye at different doses	24 and 48 weeks
Change from baseline in central retinal thickness (CRT)	Change from baseline in central retinal thickness (CRT) as measured by optical coherence tomography (OCT) in the study eye at different doses	24 and 48 weeks
Change from baseline in the annualized rate of supplemental injections	Change from baseline in the number of anti-VEGF injections which is annualized to a per year rate in the study eye at different doses	48 weeks

General Publications
No publications available

China

Recruiting

VEGFA-Targeting Gene Therapy to Treat Retinal and Choroidal Neovascularization Diseases

ClinicalTrials.gov ID NCT05099094

Sponsor Shanghai BDgene Co., Ltd.
Information provided by Shanghai BDgene Co., Ltd. (Responsible Party)
Last Update Posted 2022-08-23

Study Overview

Brief Summary
Patients who respond to anti-VEGF therapy but with refractory retinal and choroidal neovascularization diseases including neovascular age-related macular degeneration (nAMD), diabetic macular edema (DME), and retinal vein occlusion-Macular edema (RVO-ME).

Detailed Description
Choroidal and retinal angiogenesis diseases are a group of diseases characterized by choroidal or retinal angiogenesis. These diseases are often correlated with the macular area, which may lead to significant visual loss. In this study, the IDLV vector is engineered to carry the VEGFA antibody gene. The gene is delivered to the RPE cells to express the VEGFA antibody which neutralizes the VEGFA activity in the posterior segment of the eye of individuals who have progressed to various forms of neovascular macular degeneration.

Official Title
A Safety and Efficacy Study of VEGFA-targeting Gene Therapy to Treat Refractory Retinal and Choroidal Neovascularization Diseases

Conditions
Neovascular Age-Related Macular Degeneration
Diabetic Macular Edema
Retinal Vein Occlusion

Intervention/Treatment
- Genetic: BD311

Other Study ID Numbers
- BD311
- Study Start (Actual)
- 2021-11-25

Primary Completion (Estimated)
2023-09

Study Completion (Estimated)
2023-09

Enrollment (Estimated)
18

Study Type
Interventional

Phase
Early Phase 1

Study Contact
Name: Yujia Cai, PhD
Phone Number: 17721291876
Email: yujia.cai@bdgene.cn

Study Contact Backup
Name: Ting Xu
Phone Number: 17721291876
Email: ting.xu@bdgene.cn
China
Shanghai Locations

Shanghai, Shanghai, China, 200032
Recruiting
Eye & ENT Hospital of Fudan University

Contact
Gezhi Xu
86-21-54237900 medcenter@fudan.edu.cn

Contact
Jiaxu Hong
86-21-54237900 medcenter@fudan.edu.cn

Eligibility Criteria
Description

Inclusion Criteria
- Patients with nAMD at the age ≥50; or patients with diabetic macular edema (DME) at the age ≥18; or patients with macular edema following retinal vein occlusion (RVO-ME) at the age ≥18
- Early Treatment Diabetic Retinopathy Study (ETDRS) best corrected visual acuity ≤63 and letter score ≥19 Corresponding Snellen vision ≤20/63 and ≥20/400)
- OCT confirms the presence of intraretinal fluid or subretinal fluid in the fovea
- Have received anti-VEGF therapy in the past and have responded to anti-VEGF therapy

- With refractory conditions: repeated anti-VEGF treatments are required due to the disease condition. When the treatment is interrupted, the disease condition recurs (OCT examination indicates increased subretinal/inner effusion in the macula)
- For patients with both eyes suffered, enroll the one with a more severe condition
- Routine blood test, liver and kidney function, coagulation index of patients is normal: AST/ALT < 2.5 × ULN; TB < 1.5 × ULN; PT < 1.5 × ULN; Hb > 10 g/dL (male) and > 9 g/dL (female); PLT > 100 × 10^3/μL; eGFR > 30 mL/min/1.73 m^2

Subjects voluntarily join the study, sign an informed consent form, have good compliance, and cooperate with follow-up.

Exclusion Criteria

- Choroidal neovascularization or macular edema induced by other diseases
- Any other factors that affect vision improvement in the study eye, such as fibrosis, atrophy, or RPE tear in the fovea of the macula
- The study eye already has severe proliferative retinopathy, such as retinal neovascularization, traction retinal detachment, etc. (only for DME and RVO-ME patients)
- Retinal detachment or advanced glaucoma in the study eye
- Implants in the study eye (except intraocular lenses)
- Received internal eye surgery within 3 months prior to enrollment
- Vitrectomy surgery on the study eye
- Received intravitreal glucocorticoid or other clinical research drugs (except anti-VEGF therapy) within 6 months prior to enrollment
- Myocardial infarction, cerebrovascular accident, or transient ischemic attack occurred within 6 months prior to enrollment
- Poorly controlled hypertension under maximum medication (systolic blood pressure > 180 mmHg, diastolic blood pressure > 100 mmHg)
- Poor blood glucose control under medication (fasting blood glucose is greater than or equal to 10.0 μmol/L)
- Women who are willing to give birth; pregnant/breastfeeding women who have received gene therapy in the past

Ages Eligible for Study
18 Years to 80 Years (Adult, Older Adult)

Sexes Eligible for Study
All

Accepts Healthy Volunteers
No

Design Details
Primary Purpose: Treatment
Allocation: N/A
Interventional Model: Single Group Assignment
Masking: None (Open Label)

Arms and interventions

Participant group/arm	Intervention/treatment
Experimental: BD311 Adults single group Administered by suprachoroidal injection. Dosage form: injection solution. Dose: 500μL. Frequency of administration: one-time injection	Genetic: BD311 • Integration-deficient lentiviral vector (IDLV) expressing VEGFA antibody

Primary outcome measures

Outcome measure	Measure description	Time frame
Treatment-related adverse events	Observe and record incidences of AE and SAE related to VEGFA-targeting gene therapy drug BD311 (IDLV expressing VEGFA antibody) administration	At multiple time points after infusion up to 12 months.

Secondary outcome measures

Outcome measure	Measure description	Time frame
Changes in macular intraretinal fluid (IRF)	The presence of macular intraretinal fluid (IRF) will be determined by optical coherence tomography (OCT)	At multiple time points after infusion up to 12 months.
Changes in subretinal fluid (SRF)	The presence of subretinal fluid (SRF) will be determined by optical coherence tomography (OCT).	At multiple time points after infusion up to 12 months.
Change in central retinal thickness (CRT)	Central retinal thickness will be measured by Optical Coherence Tomography (OCT)	At multiple time points after infusion up to 12 months.
Changes in the area of choroidal neovascularization	Using fluorescein angiography (FFA) and indocyanine green angiography (ICGA) to assess the areas of choroidal neovascularization. Only for patients with nAMD	At multiple time points after infusion up to 12 months.
Changes in the area of fluorescein leakage	Using fluorescein angiography (FFA) and indocyanine green angiography (ICGA) to assess the areas of fluorescein leakage. Only for patients with nAMD	At multiple time points after infusion up to 12 months
The number of rescue treatments	Rescue treatments that require vitreous anti-VEGF injections due to illness	At multiple timepoints after infusion up to 12 months
Evaluate the visual improvement	Subjects will be examined for best-corrected visual acuity (BCVA)	At multiple time points after infusion up to 12 months

Sponsor
Shanghai BDgene Co., Ltd.

Collaborators

- Eye & ENT Hospital of Fudan University

Investigators

- Study Director: Gezhi Xu, Dr, Eye & ENT Hospital of Fudan University

General Publications
No publications available

China

Not Yet Recruiting

An Exploratory Clinical Trial Evaluating LX109 Gene Therapy in Patients with nAMD

ClinicalTrials.gov ID NCT06022744

Sponsor Shanghai General Hospital, Shanghai Jiao Tong University School of Medicine
Information provided by Xiaodong Sun, Shanghai General Hospital, Shanghai Jiao Tong University School of Medicine (Responsible Party)
Last Update Posted 2023-09-05

Study Overview

Brief Summary
To evaluate the safety and tolerability of intravitreal injection of LX109 in patients with nAMD.

Detailed Description
In this study, 9–12 participants were enrolled in an open monocular, single dose escalation study design. Two dose groups were set up: low dose group (7 × 109 VG/eye, 0.05 ml) and high dose group (3.5 × 1010 VG/eye, 0.05 ml). Among them, 3–6 subjects were enrolled in low-dose group and 6 subjects were enrolled in high-dose group.

Official Title
An Exploratory Clinical Trial Evaluating LX109 Gene Therapy in Patients with Neovascular Age-Related Macular Degeneration (nAMD)

Conditions
To Evaluate the Safety and Tolerability of Intravitreal Injection of LX109 in Patients With nAMD

Intervention/Treatment
- Drug: LX109

Other Study ID Numbers
- SHGH-LX109

Study Start (Estimated)
2023-09-01

Primary Completion (Estimated)
2025-09-30

Study Completion (Estimated)
2027-09-30

Enrollment (Estimated)
12

Study Type
Interventional

Phase
Not Applicable

No location data

Eligibility Criteria
Description

Inclusion Criteria
- Informed consent must be signed before all assessments
- Male or female patients ≥50 years of age
- To investigate the presence of active CNV secondary to nAMD (occult or micro-menorrhea) in the eye
- When studying the baseline of the eye, use the ETDRS eye chart to test the BCVA of 19–73 letters (approximately equivalent to decimal notation) Recorded visual acuity 0.05–0.5)
- Study eyes received at least 2 anti-VEGF treatments within 6 months. Note: For all subjects, only one eye was used as the "study eye" (i.e., the study eye receiving treatment). If both eyes of the subject meet the inclusion criteria, the eye with poor baseline vision will be selected as the study eye, or the eye with better vision may be selected for medical reasons or ethical requirements

Exclusion Criteria
- In the investigator's judgment, concomitant eye diseases of the study eye at screening or baseline may cause subjects to fail to respond to study therapy or confuse the interpretation of study findings. For example, diabetic retinopathy, retinal vein obstruction, retinal detachment, macular hiatus (stage 3 or 4), uveitis, vitreous macular traction affecting central vision, macular anterior membrane involving macular fovea or damaging macular structure, equivalent spherical lens ≤-8.00D of the study eye, etc.

- To investigate the presence of subretinal hyperreflective substance (SHRM) involving the fovea except CNV lesions
- Central serous chorioretinopathy (CSC) was confirmed in the study eyes at any time
- Study retinal detachment in the eye at any time
- Nonstudy eye BCVA less than decimal recorded visual acuity 0.05(<19 ETDRS letters)
- The presence of uncontrolled glaucoma (defined as intraocular pressure $\geq$ 25 mmHg after standard treatment) in the study eye
- Active intraocular or periocular inflammation or infection in the study eye or nonstudy eye
- To investigate the presence of CNV or macular edema secondary to causes other than AMD
- In the study, the refractive medium of the eye is seriously cloudy or the pupil cannot be sufficiently dilated, affecting BCVA or causing insufficient acquisition. Clear eye imaging data, such as OCT, FFA, and fundus photography, affect researchers' observation of safety and efficacy

Eye Treatment

- Internal eye surgery, such as vitrectomy, cataract phacoemulsification, trabeculectomy, or other filtering surgery, was performed within 3 months prior to baseline screening or study eye screening
- Study eyes screened or treated with intravitreal drug injections or drug-containing intraocular implants other than anti-VEGF drugs, such as intraocular corticosteroids, within 6 months prior to baseline
- Research eye or systemic have received gene therapy
- Study eyes screened or treated with macular laser photocoagulation or photodynamic therapy (PDT) or full vision membrane laser photocoagulation within 3 months prior to baseline;
- Study eyes were screened or underwent YAG laser posterior capsulectomy or laser trabeculectomy or laser iridectomy within 1 month prior to baseline

Ages Eligible for Study
50 Years and older (Adult, Older Adult)

Sexes Eligible for Study
All

Accepts Healthy Volunteers
No

Design Details
Primary Purpose: Treatment
Allocation: N/A
Interventional Model: Single Group Assignment
Masking: None (Open Label)

Arms and interventions

Participant group/arm	Intervention/treatment
Experimental: LX109	Drug: LX109 • LX109 gene injection Specification: 0.2 ml/bottle, 1.4 × 1012VG/ml Administration route: intravitreal injection, injection volume 0.05 ml/eye

Primary outcome measures

Outcome measure	Measure description	Time frame
Adverse Event		4 weeks

Secondary outcome measures

Outcome measure	Measure description	Time frame
Change of mean BCVA score on the ETDRS visual acuity scale from baseline	Changes of BCVA scores on the ETDRS visual acuity chart of the study eye from baseline at 4, 24, and 52 weeks after treatment with LX109	4 weeks, 24 weeks, 52 weeks
Changes in mean eye CST from baseline at 4, 24, and 52 weeks after LX109 treatment were studied		4 weeks, 24 weeks, 52 weeks
The time after LX109 treatment to the first salvage treatment		52 weeks
Proportion of subjects receiving salvage treatment in the study eye at 24 weeks and 52 weeks after treatment with LX109		24 weeks, 52 weeks
The number of times the eye received salvage treatment at 24 weeks and 52 weeks after treatment with LX109 was studied		24 weeks, 52 weeks

Sponsor

Shanghai General Hospital, Shanghai Jiao Tong University School of Medicine

Collaborators

No information provided

Investigators

No information provided

General Publications

- Wong WL, Su X, Li X, Cheung CM, Klein R, Cheng CY, Wong TY. Global prevalence of age-related macular degeneration and disease burden projection for 2020 and 2040: a systematic review and meta-analysis. Lancet Glob Health. 2014 Feb;2(2):e106-16. https://doi.org/10.1016/S2214-109X(13)70145-1. Epub 2014 Jan 3.
- Yang K, Liang YB, Gao LQ, Peng Y, Shen R, Duan XR, Friedman DS, Sun LP, Mitchell P, Wang NL, Wong TY, Wang JJ. Prevalence of age-related macular degeneration in a rural Chinese population: the Handan Eye Study. Ophthalmology.

2011 Jul;118(7):1395–401. https://doi.org/10.1016/j.ophtha.2010.12.030. Epub 2011 Mar 27.

- Ye H, Zhang Q, Liu X, Cai X, Yu W, Yu S, Wang T, Lu W, Li X, Jin H, Hu Y, Kang X, Zhao P. Prevalence of age-related macular degeneration in an elderly urban chinese population in China: the Jiangning Eye Study. Invest Ophthalmol Vis Sci. 2014 Sep 4;55(10):6374–80. https://doi.org/10.1167/iovs.14-14899.
- van Lookeren Campagne M, LeCouter J, Yaspan BL, Ye W. Mechanisms of age-related macular degeneration and therapeutic opportunities. J Pathol. 2014 Jan;232(2):151–64. https://doi.org/10.1002/path.4266.
- Mitchell P, Liew G, Gopinath B, Wong TY. Age-related macular degeneration. Lancet. 2018 Sep 29;392(10153):1147–1159. https://doi.org/10.1016/S0140-6736(18)31550-2.
- Khandhadia S, Cherry J, Lotery AJ. Age-related macular degeneration. Adv Exp Med Biol. 2012;724:15–36. https://doi.org/10.1007/978-1-4614-0653-2_2.
- Fleckenstein M, Keenan TDL, Guymer RH, Chakravarthy U, Schmitz-Valckenberg S, Klaver CC, Wong WT, Chew EY. Age-related macular degeneration. Nat Rev Dis Primers. 2021 May 6;7(1):31. https://doi.org/10.1038/s41572-021-00265-2.
- Holz FG, Tadayoni R, Beatty S, Berger A, Cereda MG, Cortez R, Hoyng CB, Hykin P, Staurenghi G, Heldner S, Bogumil T, Heah T, Sivaprasad S. Multi-country real-life experience of anti-vascular endothelial growth factor therapy for wet age-related macular degeneration. Br J Ophthalmol. 2015 Feb;99(2):220–6. https://doi.org/10.1136/bjophthalmol-2014-305327. Epub 2014 Sep 5.
- Cabral T, Lima LH, Mello LGM, Polido J, Correa EP, Oshima A, Duong J, Serracarbassa P, Regatieri CV, Mahajan VB, Belfort R Jr. Bevacizumab Injection in Patients with Neovascular Age-Related Macular Degeneration Increases Angiogenic Biomarkers. Ophthalmol Retina. 2018 Jan;2(1):31–37. https://doi.org/10.1016/j.oret.2017.04.004.

Chapter 5
Other Trials

United States

Recruiting

Microcurrent Stimulation Therapy for Nonexudative Age-Related Macular Degeneration (i-SIGHT)

ClinicalTrials.gov ID NCT05447650

Sponsor i-Lumen Scientific, Inc.
Information provided by i-Lumen Scientific, Inc. (Responsible Party)
Last Update Posted 2023-05-10

Study Overview

Brief Summary
Evaluate the safety and efficacy of transpalpebral microcurrent stimulation (MCS) therapy for patients with nonexudative (dry) age-related macular degeneration (AMD).

Detailed Description
The i-Lumen (TM) AMD device is for in-office therapy use to deliver microcurrent electrical stimulation transpalpebrally (via the eyelid) for use by an ophthalmologist. The i-Lumen AMD device contains proprietary software with preset treatment algorithms and is calibrated at each session to the individual participant.

Up to 30 enrolled participants will be randomized (2:1 active to sham ratio) and complete the initial 5-day loading treatment sessions. Participants completing the initial loading sessions will receive two (2) days of maintenance treatments and be followed through the one (1) year time point.

J. N. Weiss, *Clinical Trials in Age-Related Macular Degeneration Treatment*,
https://doi.org/10.1007/978-3-031-58803-7_5

Official Title
Microcurrent Stimulation Therapy for Nonexudative Age-Related Macular Degeneration (i-SIGHT): A Multicenter, Randomized, Sham-Controlled, Feasibility Device Trial

Conditions
Age-Related Macular Degeneration
Dry Age-Related Macular Degeneration
Nonexudative Age-Related Macular Degeneration

Intervention/Treatment
- Device: i-Lumen (TM) AMD
- Device: i-Lumen (TM) AMD Sham

Other Study ID Numbers
- ILS-AMD-201

Study Start (Actual)
2022-04-12

Primary Completion (Estimated)
2024-03

Study Completion (Estimated)
2024-03

Enrollment (Estimated)
60

Study Type
Interventional

Phase
Not Applicable

Study Contact
Name: Meredith Mundy
Phone Number: 408-440-7049
Email: clinical@i-lumen.com
United States
Arizona Locations

Phoenix, Arizona, United States, 85020
Recruiting
Associated Retina Consultants

Contact
Hannah Brookins
602-242-4928 hannah.brookins@doctrials.com

Contact
Gabrielle Santor
602-242-492 gabrielle.santor@doctrials.com
Principal Investigator:
Benjamin Bakall, MD

California Locations

Walnut Creek, California, United States, 94598
Recruiting
Bay Area Retina Associates

Contact
Luis Monslave
925-945-6800 lmonsalve@bayarearetina.com
Principal Investigator:
Caesar Luo, MD

Illinois Locations

Lemont, Illinois, United States, 60439
Recruiting
University Retina and Macula Associates, PC

Contact
Maggie Barcewicz
708-765-4110 maggieb@uretina.com
Principal Investigator:
Veeral Sheth, MD

Pennsylvania Locations

Chambersburg, Pennsylvania, United States, 21740
Active, not recruiting
Cumberland Valley Retina Consultants

Erie, Pennsylvania, United States, 16507
Recruiting
Erie Retina Research, LLC

Contact
Zoraida Santiago
814-456-4241 ext 5401 Zsantiago@erieretinaresearch.com
Principal Investigator:
David Almeida, MD, PHD

Tennessee Locations

Germantown, Tennessee, United States, 38138
Recruiting
Charles Retina Institute

Contact
Kendall Beasley
901-767-4499 kbeasley@charlesretina.com

Contact
Molly Scott
(901) 767-4499 mscott@charlesretina.com
Principal Investigator:
Stephen Huddleston, MD

Eligibility Criteria
Description

Key Inclusion Criteria
- Age $\geq$ 50 years
- Nonexudative age-related macular degeneration defined as AREDS category 3 Intermediate AMD and/or geographic atrophy
- Best-corrected distance visual acuity 20/40 to 20/200 (inclusive) in the study eye, and BCVA 20/100 or better in the fellow eye

Key Exclusion Criteria
- History and/or evidence of exudative age-related macular degeneration in either eye
- History and/or evidence of diabetic retinopathy in either eye
- Current tobacco or tobacco-related product use or history within the past 10 years of heavy smoking (on average, more than half a pack of cigarettes per day)
- Central chorioretinal atrophy in the study eye
- Glaucoma in the study eye

Ages Eligible for Study
50 Years and older (Adult, Older Adult)

Sexes Eligible for Study
All

Accepts Healthy Volunteers
No

Design Details
Primary Purpose: Other
Allocation: Randomized
Interventional Model: Parallel Assignment
Masking: Quadruple (Participant Care Provider Investigator Outcomes Assessor)

Arms and interventions

Participant group/arm	Intervention/treatment
Experimental: i-Lumen AMD Active Active transpalpebral microcurrent stimulation therapy	Device: i-Lumen (TM) AMD • Transpalpebral microcrurrent stimulation
Sham Comparator: i-Lumen AMD Sham Sham transpalpebral microcurrent stimulation therapy	Device: i-Lumen (TM) AMD Sham • Transpalpebral sham stimulation

Primary outcome measures

Outcome measure	Measure description	Time frame
Adverse Device Effects	Incidence of device- and/or treatment-related serious adverse events (SAEs) and/or serious adverse device effects (SADE) at any point during the study	Through study completion, Month 12 timepoint

Other outcome measures

Sponsor
i-Lumen Scientific, Inc.

Collaborators
No information provided

Investigators
- Study Director: Meredith Mundy, i-Lumen Scientific, Inc.

Outcome measure	Measure description	Time frame
Mean change best-corrected distance visual acuity	Mean change from baseline of best-corrected distance visual acuity (CDVA) letter score	Through Month 12 timepoint

General Publications
No publications available

United States

Recruiting

A Masked, Placebo-Controlled Study to Assess Iptacopan in Age-Related Macular Degeneration

ClinicalTrials.gov ID NCT05230537

Sponsor Novartis Pharmaceuticals
Information provided by Novartis (Novartis Pharmaceuticals) (Responsible Party)
Last Update Posted 2023-07-21

Study Overview

Brief Summary
The purpose of this study is to assess the effect of Iptacopan to prevent conversion of early or intermediate age-related macular degeneration (AMD) eyes to new incomplete retinal pigment epithelium and outer retinal atrophy (iRORA) or late AMD.

Detailed Description
This is a multicenter, randomized, participant and investigator-masked, placebo-controlled, proof-of-concept study to assess the safety and efficacy of Iptacopan (LNP023) in participants with early to intermediate age-related macular degeneration in one eye and neovascular age-related macular degeneration in the other eye. All enrolled participants must have early/intermediate AMD in one eye, with at least one high-risk optical coherence tomography (OCT) feature (study eye) and neovascular AMD in the other eye (fellow eye).

Participants who meet all of the eligibility criteria will be randomized at the Baseline/Day 1 visit in a 1:1 ratio into one of two treatment arms:

- Iptacopan (LNP023) oral capsules
- Placebo oral capsules. Approximately 146 participants (73 per arm) will be treated worldwide

Official Title
A Randomized, Participant and Investigator Masked, Placebo-Controlled, Multicenter, Proof-of-Concept Study to Assess the Safety and Efficacy of LNP023 (Iptacopan) in Patients with Early and Intermediate Age-Related Macular Degeneration

Conditions
Age-Related Macular Degeneration

Intervention/Treatment
- Drug: Iptacopan (LNP023)
- Drug: Placebo

Other Study ID Numbers
- CLNP023E12201
- 2021-001797-31 (EudraCT Number)

Study Start (Actual)
2022-02-17

Primary Completion (Estimated)
2026-09-02

Study Completion (Estimated)
2026-09-03

Enrollment (Estimated)
146

Study Type
Interventional

Phase
Phase 2

Study Contact
Name: Novartis Pharmaceuticals
Phone Number: 1-888-669-6682
Email: novartis.email@novartis.com

Study Contact Backup
Name: Novartis Pharmaceuticals
Phone Number: +41613241111
United States
California Locations

Rancho Cordova, California, United States, 95670
Recruiting
Novartis Investigative Site

Sacramento, California, United States, 95841
Recruiting
Novartis Investigative Site

Colorado Locations

Durango, Colorado, United States, 81303
Recruiting
Novartis Investigative Site

Florida Locations

Coral Springs, Florida, United States, 33067
Recruiting
Novartis Investigative Site

Saint Petersburg, Florida, United States, 33711
Recruiting
Novartis Investigative Site

Indiana Locations

Indianapolis, Indiana, United States, 46280
Recruiting
Novartis Investigative Site

Massachusetts Locations

Boston, Massachusetts, United States, 02114
Recruiting
Novartis Investigative Site

Pennsylvania Locations

Kingston, Pennsylvania, United States, 18704
Recruiting
Novartis Investigative Site

Texas Locations

Austin, Texas, United States, 78793
Recruiting
Novartis Investigative Site

Dallas, Texas, United States, 75231
Recruiting
Novartis Investigative Site

Fort Worth, Texas, United States, 76104
Recruiting
Novartis Investigative Site

Houston, Texas, United States, 77030
Recruiting
Novartis Investigative Site

China

Shanghai, China, 200080
Recruiting
Novartis Investigative Site

Heilongjiang Locations

Harbin City, Heilongjiang, China, 150000
Recruiting
Novartis Investigative Site

Tianjin Locations

Tianjin, Tianjin, China, 300020
Recruiting
Novartis Investigative Site

Puerto Rico

Arecibo, Puerto Rico, 00612
Recruiting
Novartis Investigative Site

Eligibility Criteria
Description

Inclusion Criteria

- Male or female participants ≥ 50 years of age
- Diagnosis of early or intermediate age-related macular degeneration (AMD) in the study eye as determined by the investigator on fundus examination
- Study eye (early/intermediate AMD eye) must have at least one high-risk optical coherence tomography (OCT) feature (as defined by a central reading center)
- Diagnosis of neovascular AMD (nAMD) in the fellow eye as determined by the investigator
- Vaccination against *Neisseria meningitidis* and *Streptococcus pneumoniae* infection is required prior to the start of the treatment with LNP023
- If not received previously, vaccination against *Haemophilius influenzae* infection should be given, if available and according to local regulations

Exclusion Criteria

- Concomitant medical or ocular conditions that could compromise visual acuity, require planned medical or surgical intervention during the study period, preclude scheduled study visits, completion of the study, or safe administration of the investigational product, including intraocular surgery, cataract, and vitreoretinal surgery in the study eye within 3 months prior to Baseline/Day 1 and the presence of significant media opacity, eye movement disorder (nystagmus), severe ptosis, extraocular motility restriction, or head tremor.
- History of clinically significant electrocardiogram (ECG) abnormalities, or any of the following ECG abnormalities at screening or Baseline/Day 1 visit:
  - QT interval corrected by Fridericia's formula (QTcF) >450 msec (males)
  - QTcF >460 msec (females)
  - History of familial long QT syndrome or known family history of Torsades de Pointes
- History of stroke or myocardial infarction during the 6-month period prior to Baseline/Day 1, any current clinically significant arrhythmias, or any advanced cardiac or severe pulmonary hypertension
- History of end-stage kidney disease requiring dialysis or renal transplant
- History of malignancy of any organ system
- History of solid organ or bone marrow transplantation
- History of recurrent meningitis or history of meningococcal infections despite vaccination
- History of immunodeficiency diseases, including a positive Human Immunodeficiency Virus test result at Screening
- Chronic infection with Hepatitis B or Hepatitis C
- History of hypersensitivity to any of the study treatments or excipients or to drugs of similar chemical classes or clinically relevant sensitivity to fluorescein dye as assessed by the Investigator

Evidence of cRORA or exMNV in the study eye based on multimodal imaging as determined by the central reading center.

Ages Eligible for Study
50 Years and older (Adult, Older Adult)

Sexes Eligible for Study
All

Accepts Healthy Volunteers
No

Design Details
Primary Purpose: Treatment
Allocation: Randomized
Interventional Model: Parallel Assignment
Interventional Model Description: This is a multicenter, randomized, participant and investigator-masked, placebo-controlled, proof-of-concept study to assess the safety and efficacy of LNP023 in participants with early to intermediate age-related macular degeneration (e/iAMD) in one eye and neovascular age-related macular degeneration (nAMD) in the other eye.
Masking: Triple (Participant Investigator Outcomes Assessor)
Masking Description: Investigator and Participant

Arms and interventions

Participant group/arm	Intervention/treatment
Experimental: Iptacopan (LNP023) Iptacopan (LNP023) oral use capsules	Drug: Iptacopan (LNP023) • oral capsules
Placebo Comparator: Placebo Placebo matched to study drug, oral use capsules	Drug: Placebo • oral capsules

Primary outcome measures

Outcome measure	Measure description	Time frame
Development of new incomplete retinal pigment epithelium and outer retinal atrophy or late age-related macular degeneration (AMD) in the early/intermediate AMD eye as determined by optical coherence tomography (OCT) and supported by multimodal imaging	OCT and other imaging will be performed using spectral domain OCT or swept-source OCT machines	Baseline/Day 1 through Month 24

Secondary outcome measures

Outcome measure	Measure description	Time frame
The incidence of ocular and nonocular adverse events (AEs)	An adverse event (AE) is any untoward medical occurrence (e.g., any unfavorable and unintended sign [including abnormal laboratory findings], symptom, or disease) in a clinical investigation participant after providing written informed consent for participation in the study	Baseline/Day 1 through Month 24

Change in Early Treatment Diabetic Retinopathy Study (ETDRS) (Standard Luminance) best corrected visual acuity (BCVA) scores in the early/ intermediate AMD eye	Best-corrected visual acuity (BCVA) will be measured using an Early Treatment Diabetic Retinopathy Study (ETDRS) visual acuity chart. The number of letters read correctly, for each eye, will be recorded. Participants at sites in some countries may conduct BCVA testing using numerical charts rather than letter charts	Baseline/ Day 1 through Month 24
Change in ETDRS low luminance visual acuity (LLVA) scores in the early/intermediate AMD eye	ETDRS low luminance visual acuity (LLVA) scores will be measured using an Early Treatment Diabetic Retinopathy Study (ETDRS) visual acuity chart. The number of letters read correctly, for each eye, will be recorded. Participants at sites in some countries may conduct BCVA testing using numerical charts rather than letter charts	Baseline/ Day 1 through Month 24
Change in contrast sensitivity (CS) scores in the early/ intermediate AMD eye	Pelli-Robson contrast sensitivity measurements will be performed using a Pelli-Robson contrast sensitivity wall chart and recording the number of correct letters read	Baseline/ Day 1 through Month 24
Change in Standard luminance manifold contrast vision meter contrast sensitivity (MCVM-CS) scores in the early/intermediate AMD eye	MCVM contrast sensitivity measurements will be performed using an automated device that uses an adaptive algorithm to rapidly measure a contrast sensitivity function in 5–10 minutes	Baseline/ Day 1 through Month 24
Pharmacokinetics—concentrations of LNP023 related to trough samples	Concentrations of LNP023 related to trough samples	Baseline/ Day 1 through Month 24
Change in low luminance manifold contrast vision meter (MCVM) contrast sensitivity scores in the early/intermediate AMD eye	MCVM contrast sensitivity measurements will be performed using an automated device that uses an adaptive algorithm to rapidly measure a contrast sensitivity function in 5–10 minutes	Baseline/ Day 1 through Month 24

Sponsor
Novartis Pharmaceuticals

Collaborators
No information provided

Investigators
- Study Director: Novartis Pharmaceuticals, Novartis Pharmaceuticals

General Publications
No publications available

United States

Recruiting

Study to Evaluate the Efficacy and Safety of Oral CT1812 in Participants with Geographic Atrophy (GA) Secondary to Dry Age-Related Macular Degeneration (AMD)

ClinicalTrials.gov ID NCT05893537

Sponsor Cognition Therapeutics
Information provided by Cognition Therapeutics (Responsible Party)
Last Update Posted 2023-10-24

Study Overview

Brief Summary
This is a Phase 2, prospective, multicenter, randomized, double-masked, and placebo-controlled 104-week study to assess the efficacy, safety, and tolerability of orally delivered CT1812 compared to placebo in participants with GA associated with dry AMD.

Detailed Description
This is a Phase 2, prospective, multicenter, randomized, double-masked, and placebo-controlled 104-week study to assess the efficacy, safety, and tolerability of orally delivered CT1812 compared to placebo in participants with GA associated with dry AMD.

Participants ≥50 years old diagnosed with GA secondary to dry AMD and who meet all inclusion criteria and none of the exclusion criteria will be included in the study. The study will randomize up to 246 participants in a 1:1 manner (123 participants per treatment group) to receive a single daily dose of either CT1812 (200 mg) or placebo across approximately 40–50 sites.

Following a screening period of up to 28 days, the total expected duration of participant participation in the study will be 108 weeks (104-week treatment period followed by a 28-day [4-week] post-treatment safety follow-up period).

Official Title
A Randomized, Double-Masked, Placebo-Controlled, Parallel-Group, Phase 2 Study to Evaluate the Efficacy and Safety of Oral CT1812 in Participants with Geographic Atrophy (GA) Secondary to Dry Age-Related Macular Degeneration (AMD)

Conditions
Age-Related Macular Degeneration

Intervention/Treatment
- Drug: Active Comparator CT1812
- Drug: Placebo Comparator

Other Study ID Numbers
- COG2201

Study Start (Actual)
2023-06-16

Primary Completion (Estimated)
2027-07-15

Study Completion (Estimated)
2027-08-15

Enrollment (Estimated)
246

Study Type
Interventional

Phase
Phase 2

Study Contact
Name: Diana Executive Assistant
Phone Number: 412-481-2210
Email: clinicaltrials@cogrx.com
United States
Arizona Locations

Phoenix, Arizona, United States, 85050
Recruiting
Phoenix Retina Associates

Principal Investigator:
Danesh Sharam, MD

Florida Locations

Deerfield Beach, Florida, United States, 33064
Recruiting
Rand Eye Institute

Principal Investigator:
Carl J Danzig, MD

Fort Myers, Florida, United States, 11735
Recruiting
National Ophthalmic Research Institute

Principal Investigator:
Ashish Sharma, MD

Winter Haven, Florida, United States, 33880
Recruiting
Center for Retina and Macular Disease

Principal Investigator:
Suk Jin Moon, MD

Maryland Locations

Baltimore, Maryland, United States, 21204
Recruiting
Retina Specialists

Principal Investigator:
John Thompson, MD

New York Locations

Farmingdale, New York, United States, 11735
Recruiting
Bay Area Retina Associates

Principal Investigator:
Roger A. Goldberg, MD

Oregon Locations

Eugene, Oregon, United States, 97401
Recruiting
Verum Research LLC

Principal Investigator:
Albert O. Edwards, PhD

Pennsylvania Locations

Erie, Pennsylvania, United States, 16507
Recruiting
Erie Retina Research, LLC

Contact
814-200-9152 hello@erieretinaresearch.com
Principal Investigator:
David Almeida, MD

Tennessee Locations

Nashville, Tennessee, United States, 37203
Recruiting
Tennessee Retina, PC

Principal Investigator:
Eric W Schneider, MD

Texas Locations

Austin, Texas, United States, 78750
Recruiting
Austin Clinical Research, LLC

Principal Investigator:
Brian Berger

Burleson, Texas, United States, 76028
Recruiting
Star Vision Consultants

Principal Investigator:
Courtney Crawford, MD

Fort Worth, Texas, United States, 76104
Recruiting
Texas Retina Associates

Principal Investigator:
Patrick Williams, MD

Eligibility Criteria
Description

Inclusion Criteria
- Age ≥ 50 years at the time of informed consent
- BCVA of 24 letters or better using Early Treatment Diabetic Retinopathy Study (ETDRS) charts
- Stable pharmacological treatment of any other chronic conditions for at least 30 days prior to screening

Exclusion Criteria
- GA due to causes other than dry AMD
- Any history or current evidence of exudative ("wet") AMD
- Retinal disease other than dry AMD
- Any ophthalmologic condition that prevents adequate imaging of the retina as judged by the study site or central reading center
- Intraocular surgery (including intraocular lens implantation surgery) within 3 months prior to randomization
- Any ophthalmic condition that will or is likely to require surgery during the study period
- Hypersensitivity to fluorescein
- Suspected or known allergy to any components of the study treatments
- History of vitrectomy surgery, submacular surgery, or any other surgical intervention for dry AMD
- History of glaucoma filtering surgery or corneal transplant in the study eye
- History of central serous retinopathy in either eye

Ages Eligible for Study
50 Years and older (Adult, Older Adult)

Sexes Eligible for Study
All

Accepts Healthy Volunteers
No

Design Details
Primary Purpose: Treatment
Allocation: Randomized
Interventional Model: Parallel Assignment
Masking: Quadruple (Participant Care Provider Investigator Outcomes Assessor)

Arms and interventions

Participant group/arm	Intervention/treatment
Active Comparator: CT1812 200 mg Drug: CT1812 Active Study Drug	Drug: Active Comparator CT1812 • 123 participants will receive a single daily dose of CT1812 (200 mg)
Placebo Comparator: Placebo Placebo	Drug: Placebo Comparator • 123 participants will receive a single daily dose of placebo

Primary outcome measures

Outcome measure	Measure description	Time frame
Change from baseline in Geographic Atrophy (GA) lesion area over 104 weeks in the study eye.	Compare the mean rate of growth (slope) in the GA lesion area in the study eye measured by fundus autofluorescence imaging (FAF)	Baseline through Week 104

Secondary outcome measures

Outcome measure	Measure description	Time frame
Safety and Tolerability of CT1812	Incidence and Severity of Adverse Events compared to placebo in participants with GA secondary to dry AMD.	Baseline through Week 104
Plasma concentration of CT1812	Measure pre-dose plasma concentration of CT1812	Baseline through Week 104

Sponsor
Cognition Therapeutics

Collaborators
No information provided

Investigators
- Study Director: Anthony Caggiano, Cognition Therapeutics Inc.

General Publications
No publications available

United States

Recruiting

Evaluation of OLX10212 in Patients with Neovascular Age-Related Macular Degeneration

ClinicalTrials.gov ID NCT05643118

Sponsor Olix Pharmaceuticals, Inc.
Information provided by Olix Pharmaceuticals, Inc. (Responsible Party)
Last Update Posted 2023-09-25

Study Overview

Brief Summary
This is a Phase 1, multicenter, open-label, single- and multi-dose, dose-escalating study of OLX10212 in patients with neovascular age-related macular degeneration (AMD). This study is composed of 2 parts: Part A and Part B. Part A is a single ascending dose study and Part B is a multiple ascending dose study. The primary objective is to evaluate the safety and tolerability of single and multiple intravitreal injection(s) of OLX10212 in patients with neovascular AMD.

The exploratory objectives are to evaluate the preliminary efficacy of single and multiple intravitreal injection(s) of OLX10212 in patients with neovascular AMD, and to evaluate the pharmacokinetics (PK) of single and multiple intravitreal injection(s) of OLX10212 in patients with neovascular AMD.

Detailed Description
This is a Phase 1, multicenter, open-label, single- and multi-dose, dose escalation study to evaluate the safety, tolerability, and preliminary efficacy of OLX10212 in the treatment of age-related macular degeneration (AMD). This study is composed of 2 parts: Part A and Part B. Part A is a single ascending dose study, i.e., participants will receive one intravitreal injection of OLX10212 at different dose levels and Part B is a multiple ascending dose study, i.e., participants will receive up to three intravitreal injections of OLX10212. Up to 48 individuals with AMD will be invited to participate in this study. The mechanism of action of OLX10212 holds promise to treat AMD by improving inflammation in the retina which is typically observed in patients with AMD. This is the first time OLX10212 is used in patients with AMD. The safety and tolerability of OLX10212 will be assessed via detailed ophthalmologic evaluations, vital signs, and clinical laboratory testing. In addition, plasma concentrations of OLX10212 will be measured and evaluations of the therapeutic effects of OLX10212 will be performed.

Part A uses a dose-ascending, sequential design to evaluate up to five doses of OLX10212, starting with the lowest dose of OLX10212 in a 50-μL injection. Up to six patients will be enrolled at each dose level. Each of the enrolled patients will receive a single intravitreal administration of OLX10212. The safety and tolerability evaluation period will encompass the first 14 days following OLX10212 administration. The effects of OLX10212 will be observed up to 24 weeks after injection. Based on the safety and tolerability evaluation, a decision will be made on whether or not to increase the dose to the next higher dose levels for the subsequent patient cohorts. Therefore, a total of up to 30 patients (up to 5 dose levels and up to 6 patients/dose level) will be enrolled in Part A of this study.

Part B of this study uses a dose-ascending, sequential design to evaluate three dose levels of OLX10212 (low, medium, and high), starting with the low dose. The dose levels for Part B will be determined after the completion of Part A. Up to six patients will be enrolled at each dose level. Each of the enrolled patients will receive a total of up to three intravitreal injections of OLX10212, each four weeks apart (Week 0, Week 4, and Week 8). The safety and tolerability evaluation period will encompass the first 12 weeks following the first OLX10212 administration (ending 4 weeks following the third OLX10212 administration), during which safety and tolerability will be assessed. In addition, the plasma concentrations of OLX10212 will be measured and therapeutic effects will be evaluated. A total of up to 18 patients with AMD (3 dose levels and up to 6 patients/dose level) will be invited to participate in Part B of this study.

Official Title

Evaluation of the Safety and Tolerability of OLX10212 in Patients with Neovascular Age-Related Macular Degeneration

Conditions

Neovascular Age-related Macular Degeneration

Intervention/Treatment

- Genetic: OLX10212 is a cell-penetrating asymmetric small interference RNA (cp-asiRNA)

Other Study ID Numbers

- OLX10212-01

Study Start (Actual)

2023-01-04

Primary Completion (Estimated)

2024-11

Study Completion (Estimated)

2024-12

Enrollment (Estimated)

48

Study Type

Interventional

Phase

Phase 1

Study Contact
Name: Kyungah Hong, MS
Phone Number: +82 31-779-8400
Email: kahong@olixpharma.com

Study Contact Backup
Name: Eunah Park, MS
Phone Number: +82 31-779-8400
Email: eunah.park@olixpharma.com
United States
California Locations

Santa Maria, California, United States, 93434
Recruiting
California Retina Consultants

Contact
Mary Lopez-Isidro
mary.lopez-isidro@californiaretina.com
Principal Investigator:
Daniel Learned, MD

Illinois Locations

Oak Forest, Illinois, United States, 60452
Recruiting
University Retina

Contact
BreAnne Kirby
bkirby@uretina.com
Principal Investigator:
Veeral Sheth, MD

Missouri Locations

Saint Louis, Missouri, United States, 63128
Recruiting
The Retina Institute

Contact
Lauren McDonald-Mueller
lauren.mcdonald-mueller@rc-stl.com
Principal Investigator:
Athanasios Papakostas, MD

New York Locations

Troy, New York, United States, 12180
Recruiting
Ophthalmic Consultants of the Capital Region

Contact
Kathy McNulty
kmcnulty@ophthalmicconsultants.com
Principal Investigator:
Robert Feldman, MD

Texas Locations

Bellaire, Texas, United States, 77401
Recruiting
Texas Retina Consultants

Contact
Jessica Cormier
jessica.cormier@retinaconsultantstexas.com
Principal Investigator:
Charles Wykoff, MD

Eligibility Criteria
Description

Inclusion Criteria

- Men and women ≥50 years of age
- Primary subfoveal CNV lesions secondary to AMD, including juxtafoveal lesions that affect the fovea, as evidenced by FA in the study eye
- CNV must be ≥50% of the total lesion size in the study eye
- ETDRS BCVA score ranging from 20/60 to 20/400 in the study eye
- Clear ocular media and adequate pupillary dilation (able to dilate the pupil to ≥4 mm using standard mydriatics) in the study eye to permit good stereoscopic fundus photography
- Retinal thickness ≥ 200 μm in the macular region of the study eye as measured by SD-OCT, and active neovascular AMD, in the opinion of the Investigator
- Willing, committed, and able to return for all clinic visits and complete all study-related procedures
- Able to read (or if unable to read due to visual impairment, be read to verbatim by the person administering the informed consent or by a family member), understand, and be willing to sign the informed consent form

Exclusion Criteria

- Any prior systemic treatment for neovascular AMD in either eye, except dietary supplements or vitamins or systemic anti-VEGF therapy, or planned use at any time during the study
- Any prior treatment in the study eye with another investigational agent to treat neovascular AMD within 6 months prior to Day 0 or planned use at any time during the study
- Prior treatment with anti-VEGF agents as follows:

  - Anti-VEGF therapy in the study eye within 4 weeks prior to Day 0
  - Anti-VEGF therapy in the study eye at any time to which there was no response, as defined by the presence of at least 1 of the following conditions: (1) persistent (plasma) fluid exudation, (2) unresolved or new hemorrhage, and (3) progressive lesion fibrosis
  - Anti-VEGF therapy in the fellow eye with an investigational agent (not FDA approved unless it is bevacizumab) within 3 months prior to Day 0 (prior treatment with an FDA-approved anti-VEGF therapy in the fellow eye is allowed at any time)
  - Systemic anti-VEGF therapy, investigational or FDA approved, within 3 months prior to Day 0 or planned use at any time during the study

- Scar or fibrosis in the study eye involving >50% of the total lesion size
- Retinal pigment epithelial tears or rips in the study eye involving the macula within 6 months prior to Day 0
- History of any vitreous hemorrhage in the study eye within 4 weeks prior to Day 0
- Presence of other causes of CNV in the study eye, including pathologic myopia, ocular histoplasmosis syndrome, angioid streaks, choroidal rupture, or multifocal choroiditis
- Clinical evidence of moderate or severe diabetic retinopathy, diabetic macular edema, or any other inflammatory or occlusive vascular disease affecting the retina (other than AMD) in either eye
- History of stage ≥2 macular holes in the study eye
- Any prior intraocular or periocular surgery on the study eye within 3 months prior to Day 0 (lid surgery is allowed if it took place at least 1 month prior to Day 0 and is unlikely to interfere with OLX10212 injection). Prior vitrectomy in the study eye, surgery for retinal detachment in the study eye, and prior trabeculectomy or other filtration surgery in the study eye are not permitted at any time
- Uncontrolled glaucoma (defined as IOP ≥25 mmHg despite treatment with antiglaucoma medication) in the study eye
- Glaucoma in the study eye requiring treatment with three or more antiglaucoma medications
- Active intraocular inflammation or history of uveitis in either eye
- Presence or history of ocular or periocular infection in either eye within 2 weeks prior to Day 0
- Presence of scleromalacia in the study eye
- Aphakia or absence of posterior capsule in the study eye (unless due to yttrium aluminum garnet [YAG] posterior capsulotomy)
- Prior therapeutic radiation in the region of the study eye or planned use at any time during the study
- Significant media opacities, including cataracts, in the study eye that, in the opinion of the Investigator, could interfere with visual acuity, assessment of safety, or fundus photography

- Any concurrent intraocular condition in the study eye (e.g., cataract) that, in the opinion of the Investigator, could (1) require either medical or surgical intervention during the 24- or 32-week study period (Part A or Part B, respectively), (2) increase the risk to the patient beyond what is to be expected from standard intraocular injection procedures, or (3) otherwise interfere with the injection procedure or efficacy or safety evaluation
- History of other disease, metabolic dysfunction, physical examination finding, or clinical laboratory finding giving reasonable suspicion of a disease or condition that might affect the interpretation of the results of the study or render the patient at high risk for treatment complications
- Participation as a patient in any clinical study or prior systemic or ocular treatment with an investigational agent within 12 weeks prior to Day 0
- Prior systemic or intraocular treatment with long-acting steroids within 6 months prior to Day 0 or planned use at any time during the study
- History of allergy to povidone iodine
- Known allergy to fluorescein sodium for injection in angiography
- Unwillingness among females who are pregnant, breastfeeding, or of childbearing potential to practice adequate contraception throughout the study. Adequate contraceptive measures include oral contraceptives (stable use for ≥2 cycles prior to Day 0), intrauterine device, Depo-Provera® (Pfizer, Inc., New York) or Norplant System® (Pfizer, Inc., New York) implants, bilateral tubal ligation, vasectomy, and condom or diaphragm plus contraceptive sponge, foam, or jelly. A female is considered to be of childbearing potential unless she is premenstrual, 1 year postmenopausal, or 3 months post-surgical sterilization. All females of childbearing potential, including those with post-tubal ligation, must have a negative urine pregnancy test result at Day 0 and every 4 weeks as outlined in the Schedule of Activities. A negative serum pregnancy test must be obtained at Screening.

Ages Eligible for Study
50 Years and older (Adult, Older Adult)

Sexes Eligible for Study
All

Accepts Healthy Volunteers
No

Design Details
Primary Purpose: Treatment
Allocation: Nonrandomized
Interventional Model: Sequential Assignment
Masking: None (Open Label)

Arms and interventions

Participant group/arm	Intervention/treatment
Experimental: Part A 94.3 μg/eye study eye treated with 94.3 μg of OLX10212	Genetic: OLX10212 is a cell-penetrating asymmetric small interference RNA (cp-asiRNA) • Clear colorless solution dissolved in 1X PBS and injected intravitreally • Other Names: –OLX10212
Experimental: Part A 235.8 μg/eye study eye treated with 235.8 μg of OLX10212	Genetic: OLX10212 is a cell-penetrating asymmetric small interference RNA (cp-asiRNA) • Clear colorless solution dissolved in 1X PBS and injected intravitreally • Other Names: –OLX10212
Experimental: Part A 471.5 μg/eye study eye treated with 471.5 μg of OLX10212	Genetic: OLX10212 is a cell-penetrating asymmetric small interference RNA (cp-asiRNA) • Clear colorless solution dissolved in 1X PBS and injected intravitreally • Other Names: –OLX10212
Experimental: Part A 707.3 μg/eye study eye treated with 707.3 μg of OLX10212	Genetic: OLX10212 is a cell-penetrating asymmetric small interference RNA (cp-asiRNA) • Clear colorless solution dissolved in 1X PBS and injected intravitreally • Other Names: –OLX10212
Experimental: Part A 895.9 μg/eye study eye treated with 895.9 μg of OLX10212	Genetic: OLX10212 is a cell-penetrating asymmetric small interference RNA (cp-asiRNA) • Clear colorless solution dissolved in 1X PBS and injected intravitreally • Other Names: –OLX10212
Experimental: Part B Low dose study eye treated with up to 3 intravitreal low dose injections of OLX10212 each 28 days apart	Genetic: OLX10212 is a cell-penetrating asymmetric small interference RNA (cp-asiRNA) • Clear colorless solution dissolved in 1X PBS and injected intravitreally • Other Names: –OLX10212
Experimental: Part B Medium dose study eye treated with up to 3 intravitreal medium dose injections of OLX10212 each 28 days apart	Genetic: OLX10212 is a cell-penetrating asymmetric small interference RNA (cp-asiRNA) • Clear colorless solution dissolved in 1X PBS and injected intravitreally • Other Names: –OLX10212

Experimental: Part B High dose study eye treated with up to 3 intravitreal high dose injections of OLX10212 each 28 days apart	Genetic: OLX10212 is a cell-penetrating asymmetric small interference RNA (cp-asiRNA) • Clear colorless solution dissolved in 1X PBS and injected intravitreally • Other Names: –OLX10212

Primary outcome measures

Outcome measure	Measure description	Time frame
Best-corrected visual acuity (BCVA)	Visual acuity using an ETDRS chart	28 days after last dose administration
Intraocular pressure (IOP)	Millimeters of mercury (mmHg)	28 days after last dose administration
Slit lamp	Anterior segment of the eye examination	28 days after last dose administration
Fundus examination	Posterior segment of the eye examination	28 days after last dose administration
Spectral-domain optical coherence tomography (SD-OCT)	Evaluation of retinal characteristics	28 days after last dose administration
Fluorescein angiography (FA)	Evaluation of retinal vasculature	28 days after last dose administration

Other outcome measures

Outcome measure	Measure description	Time frame
Spectral-domain optical coherence tomography	Changes in retinal thickness and relative changes (%) in CNV lesion area (mm2)	Week 24 for Part A and Week 32 for Part B
Fluorescein angiography	Changes in retinal fluid and relative changes (%) in CNV lesion area (mm^2)	Week 24 for Part A and Week 32 for Part B
Cmax	Peak plasma concentration of OLX10212	Day 0, Day 1, Day 2, and Day 3 for Part A and Day 0, Day 1, Day 2, Day 3, Day 28, Day 29, Day 30, Day 56, Day 57, Day 58, and Day 59 for Part B
Tmax	Time at which Cmax occurs	Day 0, Day 1, Day 2, and Day 3 for Part A and Day 0, Day 1, Day 2, Day 3, Day 28, Day 29, Day 30, Day 56, Day 57, Day 58, and Day 59 for Part B
AUC	Total area of plasma concentration of OLX10212	Day 0, Day 1, Day 2, and Day 3 for Part A and Day 0, Day 1, Day 2, Day 3, Day 28, Day 29, Day 30, Day 56, Day 57, Day 58, and Day 59 for Part B

Sponsor

Olix Pharmaceuticals, Inc.

Collaborators

- Trial Runners, LLC

Investigators
- Study Director: Alexander Neumeister, MD, Olix Pharmaceuticals, Inc.

General Publications
- Hwang J, Chang C, Kim JH, Oh CT, Lee HN, Lee C, Oh D, Lee C, Kim B, Hong SW, Lee DK. Development of Cell-Penetrating Asymmetric Interfering RNA Targeting Connective Tissue Growth Factor. J Invest Dermatol. 2016 Nov;136(11):2305–2313. https://doi.org/10.1016/j.jid.2016.06.626. Epub 2016 Jul 15.

United States

Recruiting

Study to Evaluate Suprachoroidally Administered CLS-AX in the Treatment of Neovascular Age-Related Macular Degeneration (ODYSSEY)

ClinicalTrials.gov ID NCT05891548

Sponsor Clearside Biomedical, Inc.
Information provided by Clearside Biomedical, Inc. (Responsible Party)
Last Update Posted 2023-09-22

Study Overview

Brief Summary
Phase 2b, randomized, double-masked, parallel-group, active-controlled, multicenter, 36-week study designed to assess the safety and efficacy of suprachoroidally administered CLS-AX 1.0 mg with a flexible dosing regimen in participants with neovascular age-related macular degeneration previously treated with intravitreal anti-vascular endothelial growth factor (VEGF) standard of care therapy. Only one eye will be chosen as the study eye.

Detailed Description
Phase 2b, randomized, double-masked, parallel-group, active-controlled, multicenter, 36-week study designed to assess the safety and efficacy of suprachoroidally administered CLS-AX 1.0 mg with a flexible dosing regimen in participants with neovascular age-related macular degeneration previously treated with intravitreal anti-VEGF standard of care therapy. Active-control will be 2 mg intravitreal injections of aflibercept dosed per the EYLEA Prescribing Information. Only one eye will be chosen as the study eye.

Official Title
ODYSSEY: A Phase 2b Study of Suprachoroidally Administered CLS-AX in Participants With Neovascular Age-Related Macular Degeneration

Conditions
Neovascular Age-related Macular Degeneration

Intervention/Treatment

- Drug: CLS-AX
- Drug: Aflibercept

Other Study ID Numbers

- CLS1002-202

Study Start (Actual)
2023-05-31

Primary Completion (Estimated)
2024-07

Study Completion (Estimated)
2024-07

Enrollment (Estimated)
60

Study Type
Interventional

Phase
Phase 2

Study Contact
Name: Donna Bezner, M.S.
Phone Number: 404.850.3421
Email: donna.bezner@clearsidebio.com
United States
Arizona Locations

Phoenix, Arizona, United States, 85020
Recruiting
Associated Retina Consultants

Contact
Study Coordinator

Phoenix, Arizona, United States, 85053
Recruiting
Retinal Research Institute, LLC

Contact
Study Coordinator

California Locations

Bakersfield, California, United States, 93309
Recruiting
California Retina Consultants

Contact
Study Coordinator

Fullerton, California, United States, 92835
Recruiting
Retina Consultants of Orange County

Contact
Study Coordinator

Mountain View, California, United States, 94040
Recruiting
Northern California Retina Vitreous Associates Medical Group, Inc

Contact
Study Coordinator

Poway, California, United States, 92064
Recruiting
Retina Consultants San Diego

Contact
Study Coordinator

Redlands, California, United States, 92374
Recruiting
Retinal Consultants of Southern California

Contact
Study Coordinator

Sacramento, California, United States, 95825
Recruiting
Retinal Consultants Medical Group, Inc.

Contact
Study Coordinator

Florida Locations

Fort Lauderdale, Florida, United States, 33308
Recruiting
Retina Group of Florida

Contact
Study Coordinator

Lakeland, Florida, United States, 33805
Recruiting
Florida Retina Consultants

Contact
Study Coordinator

Pensacola, Florida, United States, 32503
Recruiting
Retina Specialty Institute

Contact
Study Coordinator

Tampa, Florida, United States, 33609
Recruiting
Retina Associates of Florida

Contact
Study Coordinator

Georgia Locations

Augusta, Georgia, United States, 30909
Recruiting
Southeast Retina Center

Contact
Study Coordinator

Marietta, Georgia, United States, 30060
Recruiting
Georgia Retina, PC

Contact
Study Coordinator

Illinois Locations

Oak Park, Illinois, United States, 60304
Recruiting
Illinois Retina Associates

Contact
Study Coordinator

Iowa Locations

Des Moines, Iowa, United States, 50266
Recruiting
Wolfe Eye Clinic

Contact
Study Coordinator

Maryland Locations

Hagerstown, Maryland, United States, 21740
Recruiting
Cumberland Valley Retina Consultants

Contact
Study Coordinator

Massachusetts Locations

Worcester, Massachusetts, United States, 01605
Recruiting
Vitreo-Retinal Associates, PC

Contact
Study Coordinator

Nevada Locations

Reno, Nevada, United States, 89431
Recruiting
Sierra Eye Associates

Contact
Study Coordinator

New Jersey Locations

Bloomfield, New Jersey, United States, 07003
Recruiting
Envision Ocular LLC

Contact
Study Coordinator

North Carolina Locations

Asheville, North Carolina, United States, 28803
Recruiting
Western Carolina Retinal Associates P.A.

Contact
Study Coordinator

Tennessee Locations

Nashville, Tennessee, United States, 37203
Recruiting
Tennessee Retina PC

Contact
Study Coordinator

Texas Locations

Abilene, Texas, United States, 79606
Recruiting
Retina Research Institute of Texas

Contact
Study Coordinator

Arlington, Texas, United States, 76012
Recruiting
Texas Retina Associates—Arlington

Contact
Study Coordinator

Austin, Texas, United States, 78705
Recruiting
Austin Retina

Contact
Study Coordinator

Bellaire, Texas, United States, 77401
Recruiting
Retina Consultants of Texas-Bellaire

Contact
Study Coordinator

Dallas, Texas, United States, 75231
Recruiting
Texas Retina Associates—Dallas

Contact
Study Coordinator

Katy, Texas, United States, 77494
Recruiting
Retina Consultants of Texas—Katy

Contact
Study Coordinator

Plano, Texas, United States, 75075
Recruiting
Texas Retina Associates-Plano

Contact
Study Coordinator

San Antonio, Texas, United States, 78240
Recruiting
Retina Consultants of Texas-San Antonio

Contact
Study Coordinator

Virginia Locations

Fairfax, Virginia, United States, 22031
Recruiting
Retina Group of Washington

Contact
Study Coordinator

Washington Locations

Spokane, Washington, United States, 99204
Recruiting
Spokane Eye Clinical Research

Contact
Study Coordinator

Eligibility Criteria
Description

Key Inclusion Criteria
- Diagnosis of neovascular age-related macular degeneration (nAMD) in the study eye within 36 months of Visit 1.
- Subfoveal choroidal neovascularization (CNV) secondary to nAMD of any lesion type in the study eye that shows total lesion area $\leq$ 30 mm^2, CNV component area of $\geq$50% of the total lesion area, and CNV must not be associated with subfoveal hemorrhage, subfoveal fibrosis, or subfoveal atrophy.
- Previous treatment in the study eye with between 2 and 4 anti-VEGF intravitreal injections for nAMD (faricimab, ranibizumab, bevacizumab, brolucizumab, or aflibercept) per standard of care within 6 months of Visit 1.
- History of response to prior intravitreal anti-VEGF treatment in the study eye.
- ETDRS BCVA of between 20 and 80 letters (inclusive) in the study eye.

Key Exclusion Criteria
- ETDRS BCVA <20 letters in the study eye
- Central subfield thickness > 400 μm or retinal pigment epithelium detachment thickness >400 μm on SD-OCT in the study eye

- Subretinal hemorrhage, fibrosis, or atrophy of >50% of the total lesion area and/or that involves the fovea on fundus fluorescein angiography and/or color fundus photography in the study eye
- CNV due to causes other than AMD, such as ocular histoplasmosis, trauma, pathological myopia, angioid streaks, choroidal rupture, or uveitis, in the study eye
- Any history of macular pathology unrelated to AMD affecting vision or contributing to the presence of intraretinal or subretinal fluid in the study eye

Ages Eligible for Study
50 Years and older (Adult, Older Adult)

Sexes Eligible for Study
All

Accepts Healthy Volunteers
No

Design Details
Primary Purpose: Treatment
Allocation: Randomized
Interventional Model: Parallel Assignment
Interventional Model Description: Participants are randomly assigned to one of two treatment groups in parallel for the duration of the study
Masking: Quadruple (Participant Care Provider Investigator Outcomes Assessor)
Masking Description: The participant, Sponsor, Principal (noninjecting) Investigator, medical monitor, study coordinator, visual acuity technician, photographer, central reading center, and central laboratory will be masked to treatment assignment for the duration of the study

Arms and interventions

Participant group/arm	Intervention/treatment
Experimental: 1.0 mg CLS-AX Suprachoroidal injection of 10 mg/mL (1.0 mg in 0.1 mL) of CLS-AX	Drug: CLS-AX • CLS-AX will be administered by suprachoroidal injection into the study eye on Day 1 and then every 12 to 24 weeks as determined by protocol-defined disease activity criteria • Other Names: –axitinib injectable suspension
Active Comparator: Aflibercept Intravitreal injection of aflibercept (2 mg in 0.05 mL)	Drug: Aflibercept • Aflibercept will be administered by intravitreal injection into the study eye once every 8 weeks (Q8W). • Other Names: –Eylea

Primary outcome measures

Outcome measure	Measure description	Time frame
Evaluations of Outcomes Related to ETDRS BCVA in the Study Eye Over Time	Best Corrected Visual Acuity (BCVA) letter score measured on the Early Treatment Diabetic Retinopathy Study (ETDRS) chart at a starting test distance of 4 meters. The BCVA letter score ranges from 0 to 100 (best score attainable). An increase in BCVA letter score from baseline indicates an improvement in visual acuity	Baseline, Weeks 4, 12, 16, 20, 24, 28, 32, and 36

Secondary outcome measures

Outcome measure	Measure description	Time frame
Evaluations of Outcomes Related to Fluid Detected on Optical Coherence Tomography in the Study Eye Over Time	Spectral-domain optical coherence tomography (SD-OCT) is a noninvasive diagnostic technique that provides high-resolution, cross-sectional tissue imaging, and analysis of structural changes in the eye during disease progression. A central reading center will provide measurements and standardized gradings of outcomes related to retinal thickness and fluid in the eye, respectively Central subfield retinal thickness (CST) is defined as the distance between the internal limiting membrane (ILM) and the retinal pigment epithelium (RPE) in millimeters in the circular region centered on the anatomic fovea with a radius of 500 microns The presence and location of intraretinal and subretinal fluid in the central subfield (center 1 mm) is graded as Absent (the best grade attainable); Definite, outside center subfield; Definite, center subfield involved; and Definite, both center subfield and outer subfields involved	Baseline, Weeks 4, 12, 16, 20, 24, 28, 32, and 36
Evaluations of Outcomes Related to Lesion Size on Fundus Fluorescein Angiography in the Study Eye Over Time	Fundus fluorescein angiography (FFA) is an invasive diagnostic procedure used to assess the anatomy, physiology, and pathology of retinal and choroidal circulation. It involves injecting fluorescein dye into a vein in the arm/hand and taking pictures as it circulates through the eye. A central reading center will provide measurements of outcomes related to the size of lesions/leakage in the eye Total area of Choroidal Neovascularization (CNV) includes classic and occult components and ranges from 0 to 42 mm^2, with 0 mm^2 being the best measurement attainable Total lesion area includes the total CNV and associated lesion components and ranges from 0 to 42 mm^2, with 0 mm^2 being the best measurement attainable Total area of leakage includes the total area leakage from neovascularization and ranges from 0 to 42 mm^2, with 0 mm^2 being the best measurement attainable	Baseline, Week 36

Evaluation of the Number of Study Drug Injections and Supplemental Therapy Injections in the Study Eye Over Time	Number of masked study drug injections and supplemental therapy injections administered in the study eye	From Baseline Through Week 36
Evaluation of Serious Adverse Events (SAEs) and Treatment-Emergent Adverse Events (TEAEs)	The analysis of serious adverse events (SAEs) includes both ocular and nonocular (systemic) adverse events (AEs) meeting SAE criteria as defined in International Conference on Harmonisation (ICH) E6 Good Clinical Practice Consolidated Guidance. TEAEs are defined as adverse events that emerge during or after treatment with masked treatment having been absent pre-treatment or worsening relative to the pre-treatment state. Investigators will seek information on AEs at each contact with the participant. All AEs are recorded and the Investigator will independently assess seriousness, severity, and causality of each AE	From first dose of masked study drug through the end of the study (up to 36 weeks)

Sponsor
Clearside Biomedical, Inc.

Collaborators
No information provided

Investigators
- Study Director: Susan Coultas, PhD, Clearside Biomedical, Inc.

General Publications
No publications available

United States

Recruiting

Safety and Efficacy of ADVM-022 in Treatment-Experienced Patients with Neovascular Age-Related Macular Degeneration [LUNA]

ClinicalTrials.gov ID NCT05536973

Sponsor Adverum Biotechnologies, Inc.
Information provided by Adverum Biotechnologies, Inc. (Responsible Party)
Last Update Posted 2023-05-26

Study Overview

Brief Summary
Neovascular or wet age-related macular degeneration (nAMD) is a degenerative ocular disease associated with the infiltration of abnormal blood vessels in the retina from the underlying choroid layer and is a leading cause of blindness in patients over 65 years of

age. The abnormal angiogenic process in nAMD is stimulated and modulated by vascular endothelial growth factor (VEGF). Treatment of nAMD requires frequent intravitreal (IVT) injections of VEGF inhibitors (anti-VEGF) administered every 4–16 weeks. ADVM-022 (AAV.7m8-aflibercept) is a gene therapy product being developed for the treatment of nAMD and offers the potential for sustained intraocular expression of aflibercept following a single IVT injection. ADVM-022 is designed to reduce the current treatment burden which often results in undertreatment and vision loss in patients with nAMD receiving anti-VEGF therapy in clinical practice.

Detailed Description

This Phase 2, multi-center, randomized, double-masked, parallel group study is designed to evaluate the safety, tolerability, and efficacy of a single IVT injection of ADVM-022 at one of two doses ($2 \times 10^{1}1$ vg/eye [2E11] or 6×10^{10} vg/eye [6E10]) accompanied by one of four prophylactic corticosteroid treatment regimens.

Up to 72 anti-VEGF treatment-experienced study participants meeting the eligibility criteria will be randomized between the 2E11 vg/eye and 6E10 vg/eye ADVM-022 doses each with 4 prophylaxis arms for a total of 8 treatment arms, and only one eye per study participant will be selected as the study eye.

Safety, tolerability, and efficacy will be evaluated for a period of approximately 1 year from baseline.

Official Title

A Multi-Center, Randomized, Double-Masked Phase 2 Study to Assess Safety and Efficacy of ADVM-022 (AAV.7m8-aflibercept) in Anti-VEGF Treatment-Experienced Patients with Neovascular (Wet) Age-related Macular Degeneration (nAMD) [LUNA]

Conditions

Neovascular Age-Related Macular Degeneration

Intervention/Treatment

- Genetic: ADVM-022
- Genetic: ADVM-022

Other Study ID Numbers

- ADVM-022-11

Study Start (Actual)

2022-08-23

Primary Completion (Estimated)

2024-02

Study Completion (Estimated)

2024-02

Enrollment (Estimated)

72

Study Type

Interventional

Phase
Phase 2

Study Contact
Name: Sharri Adams-Edwards
Phone Number: (650) 649-1373
Email: LUNA-Clinops@adverum.com

Study Contact Backup
Name: Adam Turpcu, PhD
Phone Number: (650) 649-1012
Email: aturpcu@adverum.com
United States
Arizona Locations

Phoenix, Arizona, United States, 85020
Recruiting
Adverum Clinical Site 178

Phoenix, Arizona, United States, 85053
Recruiting
Adverum Clinical Site 126

Tucson, Arizona, United States, 85704
Recruiting
Adverum Clinical Site 159

California Locations

Beverly Hills, California, United States, 90211
Recruiting
Adverum Clinical Site 100

Encino, California, United States, 91436
Recruiting
Adverum Clinical Site 172

Fullerton, California, United States, 92835
Recruiting
Adverum Clinical Site 169

Pasadena, California, United States, 91105
Recruiting
Adverum Clinical Site 170

Poway, California, United States, 92064
Recruiting
Adverum Clinical Site 174

Riverside, California, United States, 92505
Recruiting
Adverum Clinical Site 164

Sacramento, California, United States, 95817
Recruiting
Adverum Clinical Site 166

Santa Barbara, California, United States, 93103
Recruiting
Adverum Clinical Site 175

Colorado Locations

Lakewood, Colorado, United States, 80228
Recruiting
Adverum Clinical Site 116

Connecticut Locations

Waterford, Connecticut, United States, 06385
Recruiting
Adverum Clinical Site 165

Florida Locations

Deerfield Beach, Florida, United States, 33064
Recruiting
Adverum Clinical Site 124

Fort Lauderdale, Florida, United States, 33308
Recruiting
Adverum Clinical Site 176

Jacksonville, Florida, United States, 32216
Recruiting
Advcrum Clinical Sitc 168

Hawaii Locations

'Aiea, Hawaii, United States, 96701
Recruiting
Adverum Clinical Site 149

Michigan Locations

Detroit, Michigan, United States, 48201
Recruiting
Adverum Clinical Site 167

Royal Oak, Michigan, United States, 48073
Recruiting
Adverum Clinical Site 161

Mississippi Locations

Southaven, Mississippi, United States, 38671
Recruiting
Adverum Clinical Site 163

Nebraska Locations

Omaha, Nebraska, United States, 68105
Recruiting
Adverum Clinical Site 177

Nevada Locations

Reno, Nevada, United States, 89502
Recruiting
Adverum Clinical Site 119

New Jersey Locations

Cherry Hill, New Jersey, United States, 08034
Recruiting
Adverum Clinical Site 146

Teaneck, New Jersey, United States, 07666
Recruiting
Adverum Clinical Site 171

South Carolina Locations

West Columbia, South Carolina, United States, 29169
Recruiting
Adverum Clinical Site 122

South Dakota Locations

Rapid City, South Dakota, United States, 57701
Recruiting
Adverum Clinical Site 144

Tennessee Locations

Nashville, Tennessee, United States, 37203
Recruiting
Adverum Clinical Site 101

Texas Locations

Abilene, Texas, United States, 79606
Recruiting
Adverum Clinical Site 123

Austin, Texas, United States, 78705
Recruiting
Adverum Clinical Site 154

Bellaire, Texas, United States, 77401
Recruiting
Adverum Clinical Site 108

McAllen, Texas, United States, 78503
Recruiting
Adverum Clinical Site 162

San Antonio, Texas, United States, 78240
Recruiting
Adverum Clinical Site 151

The Woodlands, Texas, United States, 77384
Recruiting
Adverum Clinical Site 107

West Virginia Locations

Morgantown, West Virginia, United States, 26506
Not yet recruiting
Adverum Clinical Site 152

France
Loire-Atlantique Locations

Nantes, Loire-Atlantique, France, 44093
Not yet recruiting
Adverum Clinical Site 502

Rhône Locations

Lyon, Rhône, France, 69004
Not yet recruiting
Adverum Clinical Site 501

Val-de-Marne Locations

Créteil, Val-de-Marne, France, 94000
Not yet recruiting
Adverum Clinical Site 500

United Kingdom

London, United Kingdom, EC1V 2PD
Not yet recruiting
Adverum Clinical Site 600

Oxford, United Kingdom, OX3 9DU
Not yet recruiting
Adverum Clinical Site 601

Eligibility Criteria
Description

Inclusion Criteria
- Male or female participants, ≥ 50 years of age
- Willing and able to provide written, signed informed consent for this study
- Demonstrated a meaningful response to anti-VEGF therapy
- Participants must be under active anti-VEGF treatment for wet AMD and received a minimum of 2 injections within 4 months prior to screening for the treatment of choroidal neovascularization secondary to nAMD in the study eye
- BCVA ETDRS Snellen equivalent between ≤20/25 and ≥20/320

Exclusion Criteria
- Any condition that could affect the interpretation of results or render the participant at high risk of treatment complications in the opinion of the Investigator
- Ocular or periocular infection or intraocular inflammation in either eye within 1 month prior to or at the Randomization Visit (Day -7)
- Uncontrolled diabetes or HbA1c ≥ 7.0%
- History or evidence of significant uncontrolled concomitant disease within 6 months of the Screening visit
- Any history of ongoing bleeding disorders or INR >3.0
- History or evidence of macular or retinal disease other than nAMD
- History or evidence of retinal detachment or retinal pigment epithelium rip/tear
- Uncontrolled ocular hypertension or glaucoma
- Prior treatment with photodynamic therapy or retinal laser for the treatment of nAMD
- Any history of vitrectomy or any other vitreoretinal surgery within 3 months prior to the Randomization Visit (Day -7)
- Prior treatment with gene therapy at any time or any nongene therapy investigational treatment or medical device in the study eye within 3 months of the Screening Visit or 5 half-lives of the investigational medicinal product

Ages Eligible for Study
50 Years and older (Adult, Older Adult)

Sexes Eligible for Study
All

Accepts Healthy Volunteers
No

Design Details
Primary Purpose: Treatment
Allocation: Randomized
Interventional Model: Parallel Assignment
Masking: Double (Participant Investigator)

Arms and interventions

Participant group/arm	Intervention/treatment
Experimental: Dose 1 A single intravitreal injection of ADVM-022 2E11 vg/eye	Genetic: ADVM-022 • A single IVT injection of 2E11 vg/eye ADVM-022 dose in combination with one (1) of four (4) corticosteroid treatment regimens
Experimental: Dose 2 A single intravitreal injection of ADVM-022 6E10 vg/eye	Genetic: ADVM-022 • A single IVT injection of 6E10 vg/eye ADVM-022 dose in combination with one (1) of four (4) corticosteroid treatment regimens

Primary outcome measures

Outcome measure	Measure description	Time frame
Severity of ocular and nonocular adverse events	Incidence of ocular and nonocular adverse events	From Baseline to Week 52
Incidence of ocular and nonocular adverse events	Incidence of ocular and nonocular adverse events	From Baseline to Week 52
Mean change in best corrected visual acuity (BCVA) from Baseline	BCVA measured by Early Treatment Diabetic Retinopathy Study (ETDRS)	Week 52

Secondary outcome measures

Outcome measure	Measure description	Time frame
Percentage of participants from Baseline who lose/gain at least 5, 10, or 15 letters in Best Corrected Visual Acuity (BCVA)	BCVA measured by ETDRS	Week 52
Mean change in BCVA from Baseline	BCVA measured by ETDRS	Week 26
Percentage of participants who are supplemental aflibercept injection-free	Supplemental anti-VEGF treatments required post-therapy	Week 52
Percentage reduction in anti-VEGF injections	Supplemental anti-VEGF treatments required post-therapy to the year prior	Week 52
Mean change in Central Subfield Thickness (CST) from Baseline	To evaluate the effect of ADVM-022 on CST	Week 52
Percentage of participants without CST fluctuations > 50 μm	To evaluate the effect of ADVM-022 on CST	Week 52
Mean number of CST fluctuations > 50 μm from Baseline	To evaluate the effect of ADVM-022 on CST	Week 52

Sponsor
Adverum Biotechnologies, Inc.

Collaborators
- Parexel

Investigators
- Study Director: Adam Turpcu, PhD, Adverum Biotechnologies, Inc.

General Publications
No publications available

United States

Recruiting

Study of Zifibancimig in Participants with Neovascular Age-Related Macular Degeneration (BURGUNDY)

ClinicalTrials.gov ID NCT04567303

Sponsor Hoffmann-La Roche
Information provided by Hoffmann-La Roche (Responsible Party)
Last Update Posted 2023-09-22

Study Overview

Brief Summary
This is a first in-human study to investigate the safety, tolerability, and efficacy of zifibancimig administered through intravitreal (IVT) injections and via the Port Delivery (PD) implant in participants with neovascular age-related macular degeneration (nAMD).

Official Title
A Three-Part, Phase I Study to Investigate the Safety, Tolerability, Pharmacokinetics, and Efficacy of Zifibancimig Following Intravitreal Administration of Multiple Ascending Doses and Continuous Delivery from the Port Delivery in Patients with Neovascular Age-Related Macular Degeneration

Conditions
Macular Degeneration

Intervention/Treatment
- Drug: Zifibancimig
- Drug: Ranibizumab
- Device: Port Delivery Platform

Other Study ID Numbers
- BP41670

Study Start (Actual)
2020-10-28

Primary Completion (Estimated)
2025-05-31

Study Completion (Estimated)
2027-03-31

Enrollment (Estimated)
251

Study Type
Interventional

Phase
Phase 1

Study Contact
Name: BP41670 https://forpatients.roche.com/
Phone Number: 888-662-6728 (U.S. Only)
Email: global-roche-genentech-trials@gene.com
United States
Arizona Locations

Mesa, Arizona, United States, 85206
Active, not recruiting
Barnet Dulaney Perkins Eye Center

Florida Locations

Saint Petersburg, Florida, United States, 33711
Recruiting
Retina Vitreous Assoc of FL

Tallahassee, Florida, United States, 32308
Recruiting
Southern Vitreoretinal Assoc

Georgia Locations

Augusta, Georgia, United States, 30909
Recruiting
Southeast Retina Center

Nevada Locations

Reno, Nevada, United States, 89502
Active, not recruiting
Sierra Eye Associates

New Jersey Locations

Bloomfield, New Jersey, United States, 07003
Active, not recruiting
Envision Ocular, LLC

Pennsylvania Locations

Philadelphia, Pennsylvania, United States, 19107
Recruiting
Mid Atlantic Retina—Wills Eye Hospital

Tennessee Locations

Nashville, Tennessee, United States, 37203
Recruiting
Tennessee Retina PC

Texas Locations

Austin, Texas, United States, 78705
Active, not recruiting
Austin Research Center for Retina

The Woodlands, Texas, United States, 77384-4167
Active, not recruiting
Retina Consultants of Texas

Eligibility Criteria
Description

Part 1, Part 2, and Part 3 Inclusion Criteria:

- Willing to allow AH collection

Part 1 and Part 2 Ocular Inclusion Criteria for Study Eye:

- Choroidal neovascularization (CNV) exclusively due to age-related macular degeneration (AMD)
- Anti-vascular endothelial growth factor (VEGF) or anti-VEGF/Angiopoietin-2 (Ang-2) IVT treatment-naïve, or pre-treated with anti-VEGF or anti-VEGF/Ang-2 no less than two months prior to Day 1
- Sufficiently clear ocular media and adequate pupillary dilatation to allow for analysis and grading by the central reading center of fundus photography (FP), fluorescein angiography (FA), fundus autofluorescence (FAF), and spectral domain optical coherence tomography (SD-OCT) images
- Decreased BCVA attributable primarily to nAMD, with BCVA letter score of 78 to 34 letters (inclusive) on ETDRS-like charts at screening. In case both eyes of a participant are eligible, the eye with the lower BCVA score should become the study eye

Part 3 Ocular Inclusion Criteria for Study Eye:

- CNV exclusively due to AMD
- Diagnosis of nAMD within nine months prior to the screening visit
- Previous treatment with at least two IVT anti-VEGF or anti-VEGF/Ang-2 administrations IVT for nAMD. The last IVT administration must have occurred at least 21 days prior to the screening visit
- Demonstrated response to prior IVT anti-VEGF or anti-VEGF/Ang-2 treatment since diagnosis
- Availability of historical VA data prior to the first anti-VEGF or anti-VEGF/Ang-2 treatment for nAMD
- Sufficiently clear ocular media and adequate pupillary dilatation to allow for analysis and grading
- Decreased BCVA attributable primarily to nAMD with a letter score of 73 to 34 letters (inclusive) or better on ETDRS-like charts

Exclusion Criteria for Study Eye

- History of vitrectomy surgery, submacular surgery, other intraocular surgery, or any planned surgical intervention during the study period
- Cataract surgery without complications within three months preceding the screening visit or planned during the study period
- Aphakia or absence of the posterior capsule. Previous violation of the posterior capsule is also an exclusion criterion unless it occurred as a result of yttrium–aluminum garnet laser posterior capsulotomy in association with prior, posterior chamber intraocular lens implantation
- Prior macular treatment with verteporfin, external beam radiation therapy, transpupillary thermotherapy, or any type of laser photocoagulation
- Prior treatment with IVT corticosteroids or implant (e.g., triamcinolone, ozurdex, iluvien)
- Subretinal hemorrhage >50% of the total lesion area and/or involving the fovea
- Subfoveal fibrosis or subfoveal atrophy
- Retinal pigment epithelial tear involving the macula
- History of vitreous hemorrhage, rhegmatogenous retinal detachment, glaucoma-filtering surgery, tube shunts, or microinvasive glaucoma surgery, and corneal transplant
- History of rhegmatogenous retinal tears or peripheral retinal breaks within three months prior to the screening visit
- Actual or history of myopia >-8 diopters.
- Uncontrolled ocular hypertension or glaucoma (defined as intraocular pressure (IOP) >25 millimeters of mercury (mm Hg) or a cup to disc ration >0.8, despite treatment with antiglaucoma medication) and any such condition, the Investigator determines if a glaucoma-filtering surgery is required during a participant's participation in the study
- Concurrent intraocular conditions (e.g., cataract, diabetic retinopathy, epiretinal membrane with traction, macular hole) that, in the opinion of the Investigator, could either:
- Require medical or surgical intervention during the study period to prevent or treat visual loss that might result from that condition; or
- Likely contribute to loss of BCVA over the study period if allowed to progress untreated; or
- Preclude any visual improvement due to substantial structural damage
- Concurrent conjunctival, Tenon's capsule, and/or scleral condition in the superotemporal quadrant of the eye (e.g., scarring, thinning, mass) that may affect the implantation, subsequent tissue coverage, and refill-exchange procedure of the PD implant

Exclusion Criteria for Fellow Eye

- BCVA letter score using ETDRS charts of < 34 letters
- Treatment with anti-VEGF or anti-VEGF/Ang-2 agents within one month prior to Day 1 (for Part 1) or prior to the randomization visit (Part 3)

Exclusion Criteria for Either Eye

- CNV due to causes other than nAMD, such as ocular histoplasmosis, trauma, pathological myopia, angioid streaks, choroidal rupture, uveitis, or central serous chorioretinopathy
- Prior participation in a clinical trial involving anti-VEGF drugs within six months prior to the screening visit, other than ranibizumab, aflibercept, or faricimab
- Active intraocular inflammation (grade trace or above), infectious conjunctivitis, keratitis, scleritis, or endophthalmitis
- History of uveitis, including history of any intraocular inflammation following intravitreal anti-VEGFor anti-VEGF/Ang-2 injections
- Prior treatment with brolucizumab
- Prior gene therapy for nAMD

Ages Eligible for Study
50 Years and older (Adult, Older Adult)

Sexes Eligible for Study
All

Accepts Healthy Volunteers
No

Design Details
Primary Purpose: Treatment
Allocation: Randomized
Interventional Model: Parallel Assignment
Interventional Model Description: Part 1 of the study will be an open-label multiple ascending dose study, followed by subsequent assignment to two groups in Part 2. Part 3 will enroll new participants to compare the efficacy of zifibancimig PD implant versus ranibizumab released via the PD implant
Masking: Triple (Participant Investigator Outcomes Assessor)
Masking Description: Part 1: Visual Acuity (VA) examiner; Part 2: Participant, Investigator, VA examiner and Sponsor; Part 3: Participant, Investigator, VA examiner and Sponsor

Arms and interventions

Participant group/arm	Intervention/treatment
Experimental: Part 1: Intravitreal Injections Zifibancimig administered in ascending dose levels through IVT injections.	Drug: Zifibancimig • Part 1: multiple ascending doses by IVT injection. Each participant will receive zifibancimig at a constant volume of 50 microliter in the study eye Part 2: participants will be randomized to one of two dose levels of zifibancimig in the PD implant Part 3: Participants will receive one of the two dose levels of zifibancimig in the PD implant • Other Names: – RO7250284

Experimental: Part 2: Port Delivery with High Dose Zifibancimig administered at a high dose through the PD implant	Drug: Zifibancimig • Part 1: multiple ascending doses by IVT injection. Each participant will receive zifibancimig at a constant volume of 50 microliter in the study eye Part 2: participants will be randomized to one of two dose levels of zifibancimig in the PD implant Part 3: Participants will receive one of the two dose levels of zifibancimig in the PD implant • Other Names: –RO7250284 Device: Port Delivery Platform • Participants will receive intraocular refillable device that is surgically inserted into the eye for continuous delivery of drugs into the vitreous.
Experimental: Part 2: Port Delivery with Low Dose Zifibancimig administered at a low dose through the PD implant	Drug: Zifibancimig • Part 1: multiple ascending doses by IVT injection. Each participant will receive zifibancimig at a constant volume of 50 microliter in the study eye Part 2: participants will be randomized to one of two dose levels of zifibancimig in the PD implant Part 3: Participants will receive one of the two dose levels of zifibancimig in the PD implant • Other Names: –RO7250284 Device: Port Delivery Platform • Participants will receive intraocular refillable device that is surgically inserted into the eye for continuous delivery of drugs into the vitreous
Experimental: Part 3: Port Delivery with High Dose Zifibancimig administered at a high dose through the PD implant	Drug: Zifibancimig • Part 1: multiple ascending doses by IVT injection. Each participant will receive zifibancimig at a constant volume of 50 microliter in the study eye Part 2: participants will be randomized to one of two dose levels of zifibancimig in the PD implant Part 3: Participants will receive one of the two dose levels of zifibancimig in the PD implant • Other Names: –RO7250284 Device: Port Delivery Platform • Participants will receive intraocular refillable device that is surgically inserted into the eye for continuous delivery of drugs into the vitreous

Experimental: Part 3: Port Delivery with Low Dose Zifibancimig administered at a low dose through the PD implant	Drug: Zifibancimig • Part 1: multiple ascending doses by IVT injection. Each participant will receive zifibancimig at a constant volume of 50 microliter in the study eye Part 2: participants will be randomized to one of two dose levels of zifibancimig in the PD implant Part 3: Participants will receive one of the two dose levels of zifibancimig in the PD implant • Other Names: –RO7250284 Device: Port Delivery Platform • Participants will receive intraocular refillable device that is surgically inserted into the eye for continuous delivery of drugs into the vitreous
Active Comparator: Part 3: Port Delivery with Ranibizumab 100 milligrams/milliliter (mg/mL) of ranibizumab administered through the PD implant	Drug: Ranibizumab • Participants will receive ranibizumab 100 mg/mL through the PD implant Device: Port Delivery Platform • Participants will receive intraocular refillable device that is surgically inserted into the eye for continuous delivery of drugs into the vitreous

Primary outcome measures

Outcome measure	Measure description	Time frame
Percentage of Participants with Ocular and Systemic (Nonocular) Adverse Events (AEs)		Part 1: Baseline up to Week 24; Part 2: Baseline up to Week 48; Part 3: Baseline up to Week 48
Percentage of Participants with Ocular and Systemic (Nonocular) AEs during Post-operative and Follow-up Periods		Parts 2 and 3: From Day 1 to Week 4 and during the follow-up period (up to Week 48)
Percentage of Participants with Adverse Events of Special Interest (AESIs) including Ocular AESIs		Part 1: Baseline up to Week 24; Part 2: Baseline up to Week 48; Part 3: Baseline up to Week 48
Percentage of Participants with AESIs including Ocular AESIs during the Postoperative and Follow-up periods		Parts 2 and 3: From Day 1 to Week 4 and during the follow-up period (up to Week 48)
Duration of AESIs including Ocular AESIs		Part 1: Baseline up to Week 24; Part 2: Baseline up to Week 48; Part 3: Baseline up to Week 48

Duration of AESIs including Ocular AESIs during the Postoperative and Follow-up periods		Parts 2 and 3: From Day 1 to Week 4 and during the follow-up period (up to Week 48)
Percentage of Participants with Adverse Device Effects (ADEs)		Part 2: Baseline up to Week 48; Part 3: Baseline up to Week 48
Duration of ADEs		Part 2: Baseline up to Week 48; Part 3: Baseline up to Week 48
Percentage of Participants with Anticipated Serious ADEs (ASADEs)		Part 2: Baseline up to Week 48; Part 3: Baseline up to Week 48
Duration of ASADEs		Part 2: Baseline up to Week 48; Part 3: Baseline up to Week 48
Change from Baseline in Early Treatment Diabetic Retinopathy Study—Best Corrected Visual Acuity (ETDRS-BCVA) Score	ETDRS-BCVA will be used to quantify visual acuity. BCVA is measured using an eye chart and is reported as the number of letters read correctly using the ETDRS Scale (ranging from 0 to 100 letters) in the study eye. The lower the number of letters read correctly on the eye chart, the worse the vision (or visual acuity). An increase in the number of letters read correctly means that vision has improved	Part 3: Baseline (baseline visit, before implant insertion) to Week 48

Secondary outcome measures

Outcome measure	Measure description	Time frame
Maximum Observed Concentration (Cmax) of Zifibancimig in Blood and Aqueous Humor (AH)		Part 1: Baseline up to Week 24; Part 2: Baseline up to Week 144; Part 3: Baseline up to Week 144
Time of Maximum Concentration Observed (Tmax) of Zifibancimig in Blood and AH		Part 1: Baseline up to Week 24; Part 2: Baseline up to Week 144; Part 3: Baseline up to Week 144
Concentration at the End of a Dosing Interval before the Next Dose Administration (Ctrough) of Zifibancimig in Blood and AH		Part 1: Baseline up to Week 24; Part 2: Baseline up to Week 144; Part 3: Baseline up to Week 144

Area Under the Curve (AUC) of Zifibancimig in Blood and AH		Part 1: Baseline up to Week 24; Part 2: Baseline up to Week 144; Part 3: Baseline up to Week 144
Percentage of Participants who did not meet Supplemental Treatment Criteria for the PD implant with Zifibancimig		Part 3: Week 40 and Week 44
Percentage of Participants who Gained or Lost ≥15, ≥10 ≥5 or ≥0 letters in ETDRS-BCVA score from Baseline	ETDRS-BCVA will be used to quantify visual acuity. BCVA is measured using an eye chart and is reported as the number of letters read correctly using the ETDRS Scale (ranging from 0 to 100 letters) in the study eye. The lower the number of letters read correctly on the eye chart, the worse the vision (or visual acuity). An increase in the number of letters read correctly means that vision has improved	Part 3: Baseline to Week 48
Change from Baseline in Central Subfield Thickness (CST)		Part 3: Baseline to Week 48
Change from Baseline Over Time in CST		Baseline to end of follow up period (up to Week 144)

Sponsor
Hoffmann-La Roche

Collaborators
No information provided

Investigators
- Study Director: Clinical Trials, Hoffmann-La Roche

General Publications
No publications available

United States

Not Yet Recruiting

Non-invasive Ultrasound Retinal Stimulation for Vision Restoration

ClinicalTrials.gov ID NCT05914233

Sponsor University of Southern California
Information provided by Qifa Zhou, University of Southern California (Responsible Party)
Last Update Posted 2023-06-22

Study Overview

Brief Summary
This clinical trial aims to test the safety and feasibility of using a noninvasive ultrasound device to stimulate retinal nerve cells and restore vision in patients with age-related macular degeneration. Previous studies have shown that artificial stimulation, such as electric and optic stimulations, can partially restore vision, but these methods are invasive and pose surgical risks.

The study aims to develop a noninvasive method for retinal stimulation. The investigators will follow the FDA guidelines to limit the ultrasound power and adhere to all clinical trial regulations to ensure all participants' safety.

The main questions the investigators aim to answer are:

- Is using high-frequency ultrasound safe using a wearable device for localized retinal neural activity stimulation?
- Does the stimulation through the device restore vision in patients with age-related macular degeneration?

Participants in this study will be asked to undergo Optical Coherence Tomography (OCT) scanning before and after the ultrasound stimulation to evaluate the device's safety. Then, they will receive five stimulation-rest cycles and complete a questionnaire to report what they see and how they feel during the device's operation.

Detailed Description
This clinical trial aims to evaluate the efficacy and safety of a new noninvasive ultrasound retinal stimulation device for vision restoration in patients with age-related macular degeneration. The investigators will take the following measures:

- The study population will consist of patients with age-related macular degeneration for whom traditional medical treatments have been ineffective and for whom there are no other viable treatment options.
- The investigators will follow the FDA guidelines and adhere to all regulations related to clinical trials to ensure the safety of all participants.
- The investigators will obtain informed consent from each participant and ensure that they fully understand the risks and benefits of the study before enrolling.

- The investigators will closely monitor each participant during the study and record any adverse events or complications.
- The investigators will use high-frequency ultrasound for localized stimulation, which is safe and effective in other studies.

Participants will receive stimulation from the noninvasive ultrasound device for five cycles and complete a questionnaire about their experiences. The researchers will analyze the results to determine the efficacy and safety of the device.

With these measures in place, the investigators believe that the study design and methodology are appropriate and will result in a low-risk study that meets the FDA's requirements for clinical trials.

Official Title
Revolutionary Noninvasive Ultrasound Technology for Vision Restoration in Age-Related Macular Degeneration (AMD) and Retinitis Pigmentosa (RP) Patients

Conditions
Age-Related Macular Degeneration
Retinitis Pigmentosa
Ultrasound Therapy; Complications

Intervention/Treatment
- Device: Noninvasive ultrasound retinal stimulation Device

Other Study ID Numbers
- HS-23-00143
- Study Start (Estimated)
- 2023-07-15

Primary Completion (Estimated)
2024-07-15

Study Completion (Estimated)
2025-07-15

Enrollment (Estimated)
5

Study Type
Interventional

Phase
Not Applicable

Study Contact
Name: Qifa Zhou, PhD
Phone Number: (213) 821-2649
Email: qifazhou@usc.edu
No location data

Eligibility Criteria
Description

Inclusion Criteria
- Diagnosis of AMD (regardless of stage and type) or RP. At least two volunteers should be diagnosed with RP.
- Age 18 years or older
- No other eye-related health conditions
- No allergic history to commercial ultrasound gel
- Must be willing and able to comply with the protocol testing

Exclusion Criteria
- Declining to participate and inability to give informed consent
- Unable to comply with the process of the research
- If the volunteer has optic nerve disease, including a history of glaucoma, optic neuropathy, or other confirmed damage to optic nerve or visual cortex damage
- Unable to fixate that hinders obtaining high-quality imaging
- High myopia; refractive error of six diopters and above
- Pregnancy
- Subject is participating in another investigational drug or device study that may conflict with the objectives, follow-up, or testing of this study

Ages Eligible for Study
18 Years and older (Adult, Older Adult)

Sexes Eligible for Study
All

Accepts Healthy Volunteers
No

Design Details
Primary Purpose: Treatment
Allocation: N/A
Interventional Model: Single Group Assignment
Interventional Model Description: Tremendous development has been achieved in the matrix ultrasound transducer. The investigators build the signal element ultrasound transducer to provide a stable energy release to stimulate a particular area. The investigators can limit the ultrasound focus to a minor point. The neuron activities induced by the focused 3 Megahertz (MHz) transducers have shown a spatial resolution of 250 ± 50 μm. According to a previous study, the Intensity Spatial-Peak Pulse-Average (ISPPA.3) is 26 (Under FDA suggestion of 28).
Masking: None (Open Label)

Arms and interventions

Participant group/arm	Intervention/treatment
Experimental: Single Stimulation of the ultrasound retinal stimulation device	Device: Noninvasive ultrasound retinal stimulation Device • Record user feelings while the device is working

Primary outcome measures

Outcome measure	Measure description	Time frame
Visual function-Assessed by Questionnaire	A questionnaire will be given to participants. The answers will be recorded as "No" or "Yes." If "Yes" is selected as the participant's answer, their descriptions according to the given questions will be recorded in detail	2 hours (average duration of procedure)
Adverse Event	The nature and number of Treatment-Related Adverse Events	From time of procedure up to 2 hours after process completion

Secondary outcome measures

Outcome measure	Measure description	Time frame
Comfort Level-Assessed by Questionnaire	A scale of 0 to 5 will be provided to the participants. 0 is no feeling, and 5 is very painful or uncomfortable	2 hours (average duration of procedure)

Sponsor
University of Southern California

Collaborators
No information provided

Investigators
- Principal Investigator: Qifa Zhou, PhD, University of Southern California

General Publications

- Ye J, Tang S, Meng L, Li X, Wen X, Chen S, Niu L, Li X, Qiu W, Hu H, Jiang M, Shang S, Shu Q, Zheng H, Duan S, Li Y. Ultrasonic Control of Neural Activity through Activation of the Mechanosensitive Channel MscL. Nano Lett. 2018 Jul 11;18(7):4148–4155. https://doi.org/10.1021/acs.nanolett.8b00935. Epub 2018 Jun 19.
- Jager RD, Mieler WF, Miller JW. Age-related macular degeneration. N Engl J Med. 2008 Jun 12;358(24):2606–17. https://doi.org/10.1056/NEJMra0801537. No abstract available. Erratum In: N Engl J Med. 2008 Oct 16;359(16): 1736.
- Chaumet-Riffaud AE, Chaumet-Riffaud P, Cariou A, Devisme C, Audo I, Sahel JA, Mohand-Said S. Impact of Retinitis Pigmentosa on Quality of Life, Mental Health, and Employment Among Young Adults. Am J Ophthalmol. 2017 May;177:169–174. https://doi.org/10.1016/j.ajo.2017.02.016. Epub 2017 Feb 22.

- Brandolin P, Martinelli G, Zanoni A. [Possibilities of use of neuroleptoanalgesic drugs of type II (dehydrobenzoperidol and fentanyl) in emergency abdominal surgery in aged patients]. Acta Anaesthesiol. 1968;19: Suppl 4:93+. No abstract available. Italian.
- Chou R, Dana T, Bougatsos C, Grusing S, Blazina I. Screening for Impaired Visual Acuity in Older Adults: Updated Evidence Report and Systematic Review for the US Preventive Services Task Force. JAMA. 2016 Mar 1;315(9):915–33. https://doi.org/10.1001/jama.2016.0783.
- TASSICKER GE. Preliminary report on a retinal stimulator. Br J Physiol Opt. 1956 Apr;13(2):102–5. No abstract available.
- Humayun MS, Weiland JD, Fujii GY, Greenberg R, Williamson R, Little J, Mech B, Cimmarusti V, Van Boemel G, Dagnelie G, de Juan E. Visual perception in a blind subject with a chronic microelectronic retinal prosthesis. Vision Res. 2003 Nov;43(24):2573–81. https://doi.org/10.1016/s0042-6989(03)00457-7.
- Ahuja AK, Dorn JD, Caspi A, McMahon MJ, Dagnelie G, Dacruz L, Stanga P, Humayun MS, Greenberg RJ; Argus II Study Group. Blind subjects implanted with the Argus II retinal prosthesis are able to improve performance in a spatial-motor task. Br J Ophthalmol. 2011 Apr;95(4):539–43. https://doi.org/10.1136/bjo.2010.179622. Epub 2010 Sep 29.
- da Cruz L, Dorn JD, Humayun MS, Dagnelie G, Handa J, Barale PO, Sahel JA, Stanga PE, Hafezi F, Safran AB, Salzmann J, Santos A, Birch D, Spencer R, Cideciyan AV, de Juan E, Duncan JL, Eliott D, Fawzi A, Olmos de Koo LC, Ho AC, Brown G, Haller J, Regillo C, Del Priore LV, Arditi A, Greenberg RJ; Argus II Study Group. Five-Year Safety and Performance Results from the Argus II Retinal Prosthesis System Clinical Trial. Ophthalmology. 2016 Oct;123(10):2248–54. https://doi.org/10.1016/j.ophtha.2016.06.049. Epub 2016 Jul 21.
- Lu Y, Brommer B, Tian X, Krishnan A, Meer M, Wang C, Vera DL, Zeng Q, Yu D, Bonkowski MS, Yang JH, Zhou S, Hoffmann EM, Karg MM, Schultz MB, Kane AE, Davidsohn N, Korobkina E, Chwalek K, Rajman LA, Church GM, Hochedlinger K, Gladyshev VN, Horvath S, Levine ME, Gregory-Ksander MS, Ksander BR, He Z, Sinclair DA. Reprogramming to recover youthful epigenetic information and restore vision. Nature. 2020 Dec;588(7836):124–129. https://doi.org/10.1038/s41586-020-2975-4. Epub 2020 Dec 2.
- Fomenko A, Neudorfer C, Dallapiazza RF, Kalia SK, Lozano AM. Low-intensity ultrasound neuromodulation: An overview of mechanisms and emerging human applications. Brain Stimul. 2018 Nov-Dec;11(6):1209–1217. https://doi.org/10.1016/j.brs.2018.08.013. Epub 2018 Aug 23.
- Liu SH, Lai YL, Chen BL, Yang FY. Ultrasound Enhances the Expression of Brain-Derived Neurotrophic Factor in Astrocyte Through Activation of TrkB-Akt and Calcium-CaMK Signaling Pathways. Cereb Cortex. 2017 Jun 1;27(6):3152–3160. https://doi.org/10.1093/cercor/bhw169.
- Chen Y, Shi Z, Shen Y. Eye damage due to cosmetic ultrasound treatment: a case report. BMC Ophthalmol. 2018 Aug 29;18(1):214. https://doi.org/10.1186/s12886-018-0891-2.

United States

Recruiting

A Study to Optimize Subretinal Surgical Delivery and to Evaluate Safety and Activity of Opregen in Participants with Geographic Atrophy Secondary to Age-Related Macular Degeneration

ClinicalTrials.gov ID NCT05626114

Sponsor Genentech, Inc.
Information provided by Genentech, Inc. (Responsible Party)
Last Update Posted 2023-10-23

Study Overview

Brief Summary
This study will evaluate the success and safety of subretinal surgical delivery as well as the preliminary activity of OpRegen in participants with geographic atrophy (GA) secondary to age-related macular degeneration (AMD). All endpoints are assessed for the study eye unless otherwise indicated.

Official Title
A Phase IIa, Multicenter, Open-Label, Single-Arm Study to Optimize Subretinal Surgical Delivery and to Evaluate Safety and Activity of OpRegen in Patients with Geographic Atrophy Secondary to Age-Related Macular Degeneration

Conditions
Geographic Atrophy

Intervention/Treatment
- Biological: OpRegen

Other Study ID Numbers
- GR44251

Study Start (Actual)
2023-03-24

Primary Completion (Estimated)
2029-04-11

Study Completion (Estimated)
2029-04-11

Enrollment (Estimated)
60

Study Type
Interventional

Phase
Phase 2

Study Contact
Name: Reference Study ID Number: GR44251 https://forpatients.roche.com/
Phone Number: 888-662-6728 (U.S. Only)
Email: global-roche-genentech-trials@gene.com
United States
California Locations

Beverly Hills, California, United States, 90211
Recruiting
Retina-Vitreous Associates Medical Group

Sacramento, California, United States, 95825
Recruiting
Retinal Consultants Medical Group

San Francisco, California, United States, 94109-5520
Recruiting
West Coast Retina

Ohio Locations

Cincinnati, Ohio, United States, 45242
Recruiting
Cincinnati Eye Institute

Description

Inclusion Criteria
- Ability to undergo a vitreoretinal surgical procedure under monitored anesthesia care
- Diagnosis of GA secondary to AMD
- BCVA score >/= 35 letters and </= 60 letters in the study eye as assessed by ETDRS
- Pseudophakic (study eye)

Exclusion Criteria
- Pregnancy or breastfeeding
- History of cognitive impairment or dementia
- Any type of systemic disease or its treatment, in the opinion of the investigator, including any medical conditions that could be expected to progress, recur, or change to such an extent that it may bias the assessment of the clinical status of the patient to a significant degree or put the patient at special risk

Ocular Exclusion Criteria for Study Eye
- Any current or history of ocular disease other than GA that may confound assessment of the macula
- History of retinal detachment

- History of vitrectomy, glaucoma-filtering surgery, or corneal transplant
- Uncontrolled glaucoma or advanced glaucoma
- Any cataract surgery or intraocular surgery within 3 months prior to subretinal surgical delivery of OpRegen
- History of other ocular or intraocular conditions that contraindicate the use of an investigational drug or may affect the interpretation of the study results or may render the patient at high risk for treatment complications

Ages Eligible for Study
50 Years and older (Adult, Older Adult)

Sexes Eligible for Study
All

Accepts Healthy Volunteers
No

Design Details
Primary Purpose: Treatment
Allocation: N/A
Interventional Model: Single Group Assignment
Masking: None (Open Label)

Arms and interventions

Participant group/arm	Intervention/treatment
Experimental: OpRegen OpRegen dose up to approximately 200,000 cells will be delivered into the subretinal space	Biological: OpRegen • OpRegen dose up to approximately 200,000 cells will be delivered into the subretinal space

Primary outcome measures

Outcome measure	Measure description	Time frame
Proportion of Patients with Subretinal Surgical Delivery of OpRegen to Target Regions		3 months post surgery
Incidence and Severity of Procedure-Related Adverse Events at 3 Months Following Surgery		3 months post surgery

Secondary outcome measures

Outcome measure	Measure description	Time frame
Proportion of Patients with Qualitative Improvement in Retinal Structure, as Determined by OCT Imaging Within 3 Months Following Surgery		3 months post surgery

Sponsor
Genentech, Inc.

Collaborators
No information provided

Investigators
- Study Director: Clinical Trials, Hoffmann-La Roche

General Publications
No publications available

United States

Recruiting

Phase 3, Randomized, Placebo-Controlled Study of Tinlarebant to Explore Safety and Efficacy in Geographic Atrophy (PHOENIX)

ClinicalTrials.gov ID NCT05949593

Sponsor Belite Bio, Inc
Information provided by Belite Bio, Inc (Responsible Party)
Last Update Posted 2023-09-28

Study Overview

Brief Summary
This Phase 3, multicenter, double-masked, parallel-group, placebo-controlled, randomized, fixed-dose clinical study is designed to evaluate the efficacy and safety of tinlarebant (LBS-008) in subjects diagnosed with GA.

Detailed Description
Subjects will be randomized in a 2:1 ratio to receive either tinlarebant or placebo. The study treatment will be administered orally once daily from baseline (Day 1) through the final day of Month 24.

Official Title
PHase 3, Multicenter, RandOmized, Double-masked, PlacEbo-CoNtrolled Study of TInlarebant to EXplore Safety and Efficacy in the Treatment of Geographic Atrophy (the PHOENIX Study)

Conditions
Geographic Atrophy

Intervention/Treatment
- Drug: Tinlarebant
- Drug: Placebo

Other Study ID Numbers

- LBS-008-CT05

Study Start (Actual)
2023-07-27

Primary Completion (Estimated)
2027-08-31

Study Completion (Estimated)
2027-11-30

Enrollment (Estimated)
429

Study Type
Interventional

Phase
Phase 3

Study Contact
Name: Belitebio Clinical Operations
Phone Number: +886 972 080 097
Email: clinicaltrial@belitebio.com
United States
California Locations

Arcadia, California, United States, 91007
Not yet recruiting
Belite Study Site

Huntington Beach, California, United States, 92467
Recruiting
Belite Study Site

Maryland Locations

Hagerstown, Maryland, United States, 21740
Recruiting
Belite Study Site

New York Locations

Westbury, New York, United States, 11590
Not yet recruiting
Belite Study Site

Oregon Locations

Portland, Oregon, United States, 97239
Not yet recruiting
Belite Study Site

Tennessee Locations

Germantown, Tennessee, United States, 38138
Recruiting
Belite Study Site

Texas Locations

Abilene, Texas, United States, 79606
Recruiting
Belite Study Site

Australia
New South Wales Locations

Strathfield, New South Wales, Australia, 2135
Not yet recruiting
Belite Study Site

Taiwan

Taichung, Taiwan, 40447
Not yet recruiting
Belite Study Site

Taoyuan, Taiwan, 33305
Not yet recruiting
Belite Study Site

Eligibility Criteria
Description

Inclusion Criteria
- Subjects must have a confirmed diagnosis of GA with atrophic lesions in 1 or both eyes
- Minimum BCVA is required in the study eye

Exclusion Criteria
- The presence of diabetic macular edema or macular disease in either eye
- Diabetic retinopathy is more advanced than mild nonproliferative diabetic retinopathy, or any other retinal vascular disease in either eye
- Uncontrolled diagnosed glaucoma in the study eye

Ages Eligible for Study
60 Years to 85 Years (Adult, Older Adult)

Sexes Eligible for Study
All

Accepts Healthy Volunteers
No

Design Details

Primary Purpose: Treatment
Allocation: Randomized
Interventional Model: Parallel Assignment
Masking: Double (Participant Investigator)
Masking Description: Eligible subjects will be randomly assigned to begin treatment in 2:1 ratio to receive the study drug (either Tinlarebant 5 mg or matching placebo)

Arms and interventions

Participant group/arm	Intervention/treatment
Experimental: LBS-008, Tinlarebant	Drug: Tinlarebant • 5 mg tablet taken orally once a day
Placebo Comparator: Placebo	Drug: Placebo • Placebo tablets for tinlarebant 5 mg prepared similarly.

Primary outcome measures

Outcome measure	Measure description	Time frame
To measure the rate of change (growth rate slope) in geographic atrophy (GA) lesion size		From baseline to Month 24]

Secondary outcome measures

Outcome measure	Measure description	Time frame
To measure the change in best-corrected visual acuity (BCVA) as assessed using the Early Treatment Diabetic Retinopathy Study (ETDRS) scale		From baseline to Month 24
To measure changes in the area and size of the inner/outer segment junction of photoreceptors by spectral domain optical coherence tomography (SD-OCT)		From baseline to Month 24

Sponsor

Belite Bio, Inc

Collaborators

No information provided

Investigators

No information provided

General Publications

No publications available

Australia

Not Yet Recruiting

Safety of BBC1501 Intravitreal Injection in Patients with Neovascular Age-Related Macular Degeneration (nAMD)

ClinicalTrials.gov ID NCT05803785

Sponsor Benobio Co., Ltd.
Information provided by Benobio Co., Ltd. (Responsible Party)
Last Update Posted 2023-10-12

Study Overview

Brief Summary
This open-label study is being conducted to evaluate the initial safety and tolerability of BBC1501 IVT in patients with nAMD. The primary objective of this study is to evaluate the safety and tolerability of three ascending doses of IVT BBC1501 in patients with nAMD. The secondary objective of this study is to exploratory of BBC1501 efficacy following three ascending dose of BBC1501 in nAMD patient.

Official Title
A Phase 1, Open Label, Ascending Dose Study to Evaluate the Safety of BBC1501 Administered by Intravitreal Injection for Neovascular Age-Related Macular Degeneration (nAMD)

Conditions
Age-Related Macular Degeneration

Intervention/Treatment
- Drug: BBC1501

Other Study ID Numbers
- BBRP11001-101
- Study Start (Estimated)
- 2023-11

Primary Completion (Estimated)
2024-01

Study Completion (Estimated)
2024-04

Enrollment (Estimated)
18

Study Type
Interventional

Phase
Phase 1

Study Contact
Name: Jihye Choe
Phone Number: +827046675278
Email: jihye.choe@benobio.com
Australia
New South Wales Locations

Sydney, New South Wales, Australia, 2000
Benobio Investigational site

Eligibility Criteria
Description

Key Inclusion Criteria

- Able to provide voluntary written informed consent on the approved ICF, understand the study requirements, and are willing to follow and complete all the study required procedures
- Male or female aged ≥ 50 years
- Diagnosed with nAMD in the study eye as confirmed by fundus fluorescein angiography (FFA)
- Active CNV lesions, secondary to nAMD as confirmed with SD-OCT (or SS-OCT), FFA, and fundus photography (FP) in the study eye
- Best-corrected visual acuity (BCVA) between 73 and 34 letters, inclusive, in the study eye using ETDRS testing
- Presence of intra and/or subretinal fluid as identified by SD-OCT (or SS-OCT) attributable to active CNV in the study eye
- Central retinal thickness (CRT) of ≥ 300 μm in the study eye as determined by SD-OCT (SS-OCT) at screening
- Participants who have had prior treatment in the study eye with any IVT anti-VEGF medication with a washout period of three months prior to the Screening visit

Key Exclusion Criteria

- Use of any of the following treatments or anticipated use of any of the following treatments to the study eye:
- Intravitreal or periocular corticosteroid, within 90 days prior to Visit 1 (Day 1) and throughout the study
- BCVA worse than 20/400 in study eye; worse than 20/200 in fellow eye
- Uncontrolled or advanced glaucoma, evidenced by an IOP of > 21 mmHg or cup/disc ratio > 0.8 while on medical therapy, or chronic hypotony (< 6 mmHg) in the study eye
- Evidence of any other ocular disease other than nAMD in the study eye that may confound the outcome of the study (e.g., active diabetic retinopathy, posterior uveitis, pseudovitelliform macular degeneration, moderate/severe myopia)

- History of vitrectomy in the study eye
- Need for ocular surgery in the study eye during the course of the study
- YAG laser capsulotomy within 30 days prior to Visit 1 (Day 1) in the study eye
- Intraocular surgery, including lens removal or laser, within 90 days prior to Visit 1 (Day 1) in the study eye
- Ocular or periocular infection in either eye
- Pupillary dilation inadequate for quality stereoscopic fundus photography in the study eye
- Media opacity that would limit clinical visualization, intravenous fluorescein angiography, or spectral-domain optical coherence tomography (SD-OCT) evaluation in the study eye
- History of herpetic infection in the study eye or adnexa
- Presence of known active toxoplasmosis, inactive toxoplasmosis, or toxoplasmosis scar in either eye
- Presence of any form of ocular malignancy including choroidal melanoma in either eye

Ages Eligible for Study
50 Years and Older (Adult, Older Adult)

Sexes Eligible for Study
All

Accepts Healthy Volunteers
No

Design Details
Primary Purpose: Treatment
Allocation: Nonrandomized
Interventional Model: Sequential Assignment
Masking: None (Open Label)

Arms and interventions

Participant group/arm	Intervention/treatment
Experimental: BBC1501 1.25μg Cohort 1; open-label, nonrandomized, single administration	Drug: BBC1501 • BBC1501 solution for Intravitreal injection
Experimental: BBC1501 2.5μg Cohort 2; open-label, nonrandomized, single administration	Drug: BBC1501 • BBC1501 solution for Intravitreal injection
Experimental: BBC1501 5μg Cohort 3; open-label, nonrandomized, single administration	Drug: BBC1501 • BBC1501 solution for Intravitreal injection

Primary outcome measures

Outcome measure	Measure description	Time frame
Assessment of ophthalmic and systemic TEAEs, during the study period	To evaluate the safety and tolerability of a single IVT dose of BBC1501 at 4 weeks after dose. To characterize ocular and nonocular safety by the incidence of treatment-emergent adverse events (AEs) (new or worsening from baseline) summarized categorically by system organ class and/or preferred term	Every week up to 4 weeks
Assessment of ophthalmic and systemic TEAEs, during study period	To evaluate the safety and tolerability of a single IVT dose of BBC1501 at 12 weeks after dose. To characterize ocular and nonocular safety by the incidence of treatment-emergent adverse events (AEs) (new or worsening from baseline) summarized categorically by system organ class and/or preferred term.	every 4 weeks up to 12 weeks

Secondary outcome measures

Outcome measure	Measure description	Time frame
Mean change in Early Treatment Diabetic Retinopathy Study (ETDRS) BCVA from baseline	Assessment of ETDRS change from baseline by Optical Coherence Tomography (OCT)	Baseline, Week 4
Mean change in Early Treatment Diabetic Retinopathy Study (ETDRS) BCVA from baseline	Assessment of ETDRS change from baseline by Optical Coherence Tomography (OCT)	Baseline, Week 12
Change in CNV size according to fluorescein angiogram	Assessment of CNV size change from baseline by Fundus fluorescein angiography (FFA)	Baseline, Week 4
Change in CNV size according to fluorescein angiogram	Assessment of CNV size change from baseline by Fundus fluorescein angiography (FFA)	Baseline, Week 12
Changes in intra-or sub-retinal fluid measured as mean change in central retinal thickness or macula volume	Assessment of Central retinal thickness from baseline by Spectral Domain Optical Coherence Tomography (SD-OCT)	Baseline, Week 4
Changes in intra-or sub-retinal fluid measured as mean change in central retinal thickness or macula volume	Assessment of Central retinal thickness from baseline by Spectral Domain Optical Coherence Tomography (SD-OCT)	Baseline, Week 12
Number of patients who initiated rescue therapy during the study	Exploratory use rescue therapy during the study and follow-up period	Week 1, Week 12

Sponsor
Benobio Co., Ltd.

Collaborators
No information provided

Investigators
- Study Chair: Inhyun Lee, Ph.D, Benobio Co., Ltd.

General Publications
No publications available

Australia

Recruiting

Subthreshold Laser Treatment in Intermediate Age-Related Macular Degeneration with Nascent Geographic Atrophy Study (LIANA)

ClinicalTrials.gov ID NCT05200624

Sponsor Center for Eye Research Australia
Information provided by Center for Eye Research Australia (Responsible Party)
Last Update Posted 2023-03-27

Study Overview

Brief Summary
This study is a prospective, single-centre, randomized, sham-controlled, double-masked, clinical trial that aims to investigate the effect of subthreshold nanosecond laser on disease progression in eyes with intermediate age-related macular degeneration (AMD) and nascent geographic atrophy by functional and anatomical outcomes.

The study population will be individuals with high-risk intermediate age-related macular degeneration who meet all eligibility criteria. Sixty subjects total (30 randomized to receive subthreshold nanosecond laser (SNL) treatment and 30 to receive sham treatment per the 1:1 randomization).

The study has a 12-month study period with four scheduled visits: screening, randomization (first treatment), 6-month follow-up visit (with second treatment where eligible), and 12-month follow-up.

The primary outcome is the proportion of laser-treated study eyes that develop late AMD compared to sham-treated study eyes over 12 months. The key secondary outcome is the change in retinal function of laser-treated study eyes compared to sham-treated study eyes over 12 months. Safety will be the proportion of laser-treated eyes that lose 10+ letters of vision (measured on a standard vision chart) compared to sham-treated eyes over 12 months.

Official Title
Subthreshold Laser Treatment in Intermediate Age-Related Macular Degeneration with Nascent Geographic Atrophy Study

Conditions
Age-Related Macular Degeneration

Intervention/Treatment
- Device: 2RT subthreshold nanosecond laser

Other Study ID Numbers
- LIANA

Study Start (Actual)
2021-12-13

Primary Completion (Estimated)
2024-12-31

Study Completion (Estimated)
2024-12-31

Enrollment (Estimated)
60

Study Type
Interventional

Phase
Not Applicable

Study Contact
Name: Carly Parfett
Phone Number: +61399298263
Email: cera-rgo@cera.org.au

Study Contact Backup
Name: Rebecca Singleton
Phone Number: +61399298369
Email: cera-rgo@cera.org.au
Australia
Victoria Locations

East Melbourne, Victoria, Australia, 3002
Recruiting
Centre for Eye Research Australia

Contact
Carly Parfett
+61 3 9929 8263 cera-rgo@cera.org.au
Principal Investigator:
Robyn H Guymer

Eligibility Criteria
Description

Inclusion Criteria
- Age 50 years or older at the time of consent
- Best-corrected visual acuity (BCVA) of 59 letters (Snellen equivalent of 6/19) or better in both eyes
- Bilateral large (>125 μm) drusen as seen on color fundus photographs (CFP) as assessed within a circle with a radius of 3000 μm centered on the fovea
- Between 1 and 5 (inclusive) discrete area/s of nascent geographic atrophy (nGA) as seen on SD-OCT B-scan/s within a 20°x20° volume scan centered on the

fovea in the study eye. NOTE: The nonstudy eye may have no nGA or any number of nGA lesions but not cRORA (on B-scan) or GA (on CFP)
- Ability, willingness, and sufficient cognitive awareness to consent to the trial, received randomized SNL treatment or sham procedure, and complete all visits as per the study schedule

Exclusion Criteria
- A cluster of definitely present reticular pseudodrusen (RPD) of >1 disc area (DA) as seen on infrared (IR) imaging or fundus autofluorescence (FAF) within a 20°x20° field centered on the fovea
- Any evidence of definite geographic atrophy (GA)
- Any evidence of OCT-atrophy greater than nGA, i.e., complete RPE and outer retinal atrophy (cRORA) as determined on a SD-OCT 20°x20° volume scan centered on the fovea
- Any evidence of active, regressed, or treated macular neovascularization (MNV), in either eye, or active peripapillary CNV in the study eye (determined on multimodal imaging and a fundus fluorescein angiogram is only required if in the investigator's medical judgement). NOTE: Subretinal fluid (SRF) <100 μm or SRF associated with a subfoveal pseudovitelliform lesion permitted (i.e., slither/draping/vitelliform with no evidence of new vessels on OCT-A) is not considered MNV and can be enrolled
- A subfoveal pigment epithelial detachment (PED)/drusenoid detachment >1000 μm in diameter (measured on the central B-scan) with hyperreflective foci (HRF) and increased choroidal transmission or any PED >2000 μm measured at the central foveal B-scan
- Any other investigational treatment for AMD, excluding dietary supplements, received in the past 12 months or thought, in the opinion of the investigator, likely to chronically change the course of the subject's retinal disease
- Current participation in any other investigational ophthalmological clinical trial
- Any ocular disease in the study eye, other than AMD, which in the opinion of the investigator may significantly compromise the assessment of the retina, or which would compromise the ability to assess any effect following SNL treatment including, but not limited to:
  - Diabetic retinopathy (unless limited to fewer than 10 microaneurysms and/or small retinal hemorrhages, without retinal thickening on OCT)
  - Macular pathology or pigmentary abnormalities atypical of AMD, including but not limited to pattern dystrophy, myopic maculopathy, angioid streaks, resumed ocular histoplasmosis syndrome, central serous choroidopathy, visually significant epiretinal membranes, macular hole, or pseudohole
  - Optic nerve pathology, including optic atrophy, history of optic neuropathy
  - Myopic crescent wider than 50% of the longest diameter of the optic disc or closer than 1500 μm to the fovea
  - Retinal vascular diseases including branch or central vein or artery occlusion
  - Choroidal nevus within 2 disc diameters (DD) of the fovea associated with depigmentation or overlying drusen, if these drusen are used to determine eligibility
  - Active uveitis or ocular inflammation

- History or the presence of uncontrolled glaucoma
- Intraocular pressure that would preclude safe dilation of the pupil to allow adequate assessment and application of SNL treatment
- History of prior laser surgery to the retina including subthreshold laser (focal retinopexy for a peripheral break and/or focal retinal tears performed more than 90 days prior to the entry into the study is permitted)
- Significant cataract or other ocular media which, in the opinion of the investigator, significantly limits the visual acuity or view of the retina
- Previous retinal or ocular surgery, the effects of which may now or in the future complicate the assessment of the progression of AMD (cataract surgery is allowed as long as it was performed over 90 days prior to entry into the study)
- Known hypersensitivity to fluorescein
- Sensitivity to application of a contact lens
- Corneal pathology precluding visualization of the fundus or increasing the risk of using a contact lens, such as corneal dystrophy, recurrent corneal erosion syndrome, or sensitivity to the application of a contact lens
- Use of any systemic or ocular medication known to be toxic to the retina, excluding tamoxifen unless there is evidence of toxicity
- Pregnant or lactating women
- Subject who is considered ineligible for this study in the investigator's medical judgment

Ages Eligible for Study
50 Years and Older (Adult, Older Adult)

Sexes Eligible for Study
All

Accepts Healthy Volunteers
No

Design Details
Primary Purpose: Treatment
Allocation: Randomized
Interventional Model: Parallel Assignment
Masking: Double (Participant Outcomes Assessor)

Arms and interventions

Participant group/arm	Intervention/treatment
Active Comparator: Active laser Application of the active 2RT subthreshold laser	Device: 2RT subthreshold nanosecond laser • The 2RT™ Q-switched YAG laser (532 nm) delivering 3 nanosecond pulses; 400 μm spot size, is a pulsed subthreshold nanosecond (SNL) laser, which uses low energy levels to produce limited effects that selectively target melanosomes within the pigmented retinal pigment epithelial (RPE) cells • Other Names: –2RT –SNL
Sham Comparator: Sham laser Application of sham laser (i.e., flashing lights that replicate the look of active laser to the participant)	Device: 2RT subthreshold nanosecond laser • The 2RT™ Q-switched YAG laser (532 nm) delivering 3 nanosecond pulses; 400 μm spot size, is a pulsed subthreshold nanosecond (SNL) laser, which uses low energy levels to produce limited effects that selectively target melanosomes within the pigmented retinal pigment epithelial (RPE) cells • Other Names: –2RT –SNL

Primary outcome measures

Outcome measure	Measure description	Time frame
Rate of progression to advanced AMD in study eyes	The time to develop advanced AMD—as defined as choroidal neovascularization (CNV), geographic atrophy (GA), or OCT-defined cRORA—in the SNL-treated compared to sham-treated study eyes over 12 months	12 months

Secondary outcome measures

Outcome measure	Measure description	Time frame
Rate of retinal sensitivity change in study eyes	The rate of change in mean retinal sensitivity over time (in decibels per year) of the SNL-treated compared to sham-treated study eyes over 12 months	12 months

Other outcome measures

Outcome measure	Measure description	Time frame
Safety Endpoint: Proportion of study eyes with a ≥ 10-letter loss in best-corrected visual acuity (BCVA)	The proportion of eyes that lose ≥10 letters of BCVA in the SNL-treated compared to sham-treated study and fellow eyes over 12 months	12 months

Sponsor

Center for Eye Research Australia

Collaborators

- AlphaRET Pty Ltd.

Investigators

- Principal Investigator: Robyn H Guymer, MBBS FRANZCO, Centre for Eye Research Australia

General Publications
No publications available

Austria

Recruiting

Faricimab for High-Frequent Aflibercept Treated Neovascular Age-Related Macular Degeneration (FAN)

ClinicalTrials.gov ID NCT05941715

Sponsor Medical University of Graz
Information provided by Medical University of Graz (Responsible Party)
Last Update Posted 2023-07-24

Study Overview

Brief Summary
Study purpose: To evaluate if previously high-frequent (3-5 weekly) aflibercept-treated neovascular age-related macular degeneration (nAMD) can be extended in their treatment interval when switched to faricimab.

Primary objective: To assess the efficacy of faricimab compared to aflibercept in terms of durability at 32 weeks by extending treatment interval in previous high-frequent aflibercept treated nAMD.

Detailed Description
There is a subgroup of nAMD patients requiring monthly interventions when applying as needed and treat-and-extend treatment strategies. A burden for both patients/caregivers and healthcare systems. More durable treatment options are needed to increase the quality of life for these nAMD patients, as well as to make human resources available for the growing elderly AMD population requiring treatment.

The FAN study is a randomized, double-masked, 2-arm (comparator-controlled), phase-IV, monocenter study with a primary endpoint at 32 weeks. The study is conducted in two parts. Patients will receive either aflibercept or faricimab via the treat-and-extend principle until the primary endpoint (part 1). As mentioned, the main objective is to assess the durability of both drugs in this particular subgroup of nAMD patients. In part 2 of the study, starting at or after 32 weeks, all patients will receive faricimab via the treat-and-extend principle until the end of the study (56 weeks).

Official Title
Faricimab for High-frequent Aflibercept Treated Neovascular Age-Related Macular Degeneration: A Monocenter, Randomized, Double-Masked Comparator-Controlled Study (FAN)

Conditions
Neovascular Age-Related Macular Degeneration

Intervention/Treatment
- Drug: Aflibercept 40 MG/ML
- Drug: Faricimab 120 MG/ML

Other Study ID Numbers
- 35-200 ex 22/23
- 2023-000037-32 (EudraCT Number)

Study Start (Actual)
2023-07-04

Primary Completion (Estimated)
2024-06

Study Completion (Estimated)
2024-12

Enrollment (Estimated)
70

Study Type
Interventional

Phase
Phase 4

Study Contact
Name: Monja Michelitsch, MD
Phone Number: 0043(0)31638513817
Email: monja.michelitsch@medunigraz.at
Austria
Styria Locations

Graz, Styria, Austria, 8036
Recruiting
Department of Ophthalmology, Medical University Graz

Contact
Andreas Wedrich
0043(0)31638513817 andreas.wedrich@medunigraz.at

Eligibility Criteria
Description

Ocular Inclusion Criteria
- MNV due to AMD (nAMD)
- BVCA between and including 19 and 75 letters (Snellen equivalent approximately 20/400 to 20/32)

- ≥ 7 previous intravitreal injections with anti-VEGF
- The last ≥ 4 consecutive intravitreal injections with aflibercept
- The last aflibercept injections within the last 35 days
- Interval between the last two aflibercept injections ≤ 35 days

Ocular Exclusion Criteria
- MNV due to other causes than nAMD
- Polypoidal choroidal neovascularization
- Retinal pigment epithelial rip/tear
- Subretinal hemorrhage of > 50% of the lesion, involving the fovea
- Any macular pathology other than AMD causing structural changes of the macula and thereby affecting vision
- Any active intra-/periocular infection/inflammation of the study eye
- Uncontrolled glaucoma under medication (IOP >25 mmHg)
- Cataract surgery of the study eye within the last 3 months
- Previous intraocular surgery of the study eye other than cataract surgery or intravitreal injections with anti-VEGF (e.g., vitrectomy, corneal transplant, glaucoma surgery)
- Any previous laser therapy of the study eye other than Yag (yttrium aluminum garnet) laser capsulotomy (e.g., panretinal photocoagulation, verteporfin photodynamic therapy)
- Refractive error of more than -6 diopters myopia
- Vitreous hemorrhage
- Retinal detachment

General Exclusion Criteria
- Use of long-term systemic corticosteroids within the last 3 months
- Uncontrolled blood pressure (either/both systolic blood pressure >180 mmHg, diastolic blood pressure >100 mmHg)
- Pregnancy (pre-menopausal women MUST take a pregnancy test at the time of initiation)
- Breast-feeding
- Myocardial infarction or stroke within the last six months
- Concomitant participation in another clinical study with investigational medicinal products
- A known allergy or hypersensitivity toward eye drops needed for the examinations planned during the study, and/or the intravitreal procedure
- A known allergy or hypersensitivity against fluorescein/indocyanine green used during angiography
- A known allergy or hypersensitivity toward any of the components of the study drug

Ages Eligible for Study
50 Years and Older (Adult, Older Adult)

Sexes Eligible for Study
All

Accepts Healthy Volunteers
No

Design Details
Primary Purpose: Treatment
Allocation: Randomized
Interventional Model: Parallel Assignment
Masking: Triple (Participant Investigator Outcomes Assessor)

Arms and interventions

Participant group/arm	Intervention/treatment
Active Comparator: group A: aflibercept first (part 1), switch to faricimab (part 2) Aflibercept 2.0 mg/0.05 ml intravitreal will be administered from baseline through to the first visit at or after 32 weeks in a treat-and-extend regime. At the first visit at or after 32 weeks, faricimab 6.0 mg/0.05 ml intravitreal will be administered in a treat-and-extend regime through to the last visit before 56 weeks.	Drug: Aflibercept 40 MG/ML • treat-and-extend • Other Names: –Eylea® Drug: Faricimab 120 MG/ML • treat-and-extend • Other Names: –Vabysmo®
Experimental: group B: faricimab monotherapy Faricimab 6.0 mg/0.05 ml intravitreal will be administered from baseline through to the last visit before 56 weeks in a treat-and-extend regime	Drug: Faricimab 120 MG/ML • treat-and-extend • Other Names: –Vabysmo®

Primary outcome measures

Outcome measure	Measure description	Time frame
Proportion of eyes with at least one extension without retinal (intra- and subretinal) fluid within the time period baseline to 32 weeks (extension success rate)	Treatment is administered at each visit. The interval between treatments is based on a treat and extend regime. The first interval between treatments, from baseline, is 4 weeks. Intra- and subretinal fluid are assessed at each visit with optical coherence tomography (OCT). Should no intra- and subretinal fluid be present on OCT, the treatment interval to the next visit is extended by 2 weeks. Is intra- and or subretinal fluid present on OCT, the treatment interval to the next visit is reduced by 2 weeks. The minimum treatment interval is 4 weeks, the maximum treatment interval is 12 weeks	at 32 weeks

Secondary outcome measures

Outcome measure	Measure description	Time frame
Proportion of eyes with maximum extended interval without retinal (intra- and subretinal) fluid of ≥ 6, ≥ 8, ≥ 10 weeks and (≥ 12 weeks)	Treatment is administered at each visit. The interval between treatments is based on a treat and extend regime. The first interval between treatments, from baseline, is 4 weeks. Intra- and subretinal fluid are assessed at each visit with optical coherence tomography (OCT). Should no intra- and subretinal fluid be present on OCT, the treatment interval to the next visit is extended by 2 weeks. Is intra- and or subretinal fluid present on OCT, the treatment interval to the next visit is reduced by 2 weeks. The minimum treatment interval is 4 weeks, and the maximum treatment interval is 12 weeks	at 32 weeks and 56 weeks
Maximum extended treatment interval without retinal (intra- and subretinal) fluid	Treatment is administered at each visit. The interval between treatments is based on a treat and extend regime. The first interval between treatments, from baseline, is 4 weeks. Intra- and subretinal fluid are assessed at each visit with optical coherence tomography (OCT). Should no intra- and subretinal fluid be present on OCT, the treatment interval to the next visit is extended by 2 weeks. Is intra- and or subretinal fluid present on OCT, the treatment interval to the next visit is reduced by 2 weeks. The minimum treatment interval is 4 weeks, and the maximum treatment interval is 12 weeks	at 32 weeks and 56 weeks
Number of injections received		during 32 weeks and 1 year
Proportion of eyes remaining on a 4-weekly interval from baseline to the last visit (completed interval)	Treatment is administered at each visit. The interval between treatments is based on a treat and extend regime. The first interval between treatments, from baseline, is 4 weeks. Intra- and subretinal fluid are assessed at each visit with optical coherence tomography (OCT). Should no intra- and subretinal fluid be present on OCT, the treatment interval to the next visit is extended by 2 weeks. Is intra- and or subretinal fluid present on OCT, the treatment interval to the next visit is reduced by 2 weeks. The minimum treatment interval is 4 weeks, and the maximum treatment interval is 12 weeks	at 32 weeks and 56 weeks

Other outcome measures

Outcome measure	Measure description	Time frame
Mean change in ETDRS letter score	Best Corrected Visual Acuity (BCVA) is measured via Early Treatment Diabetic Retinopathy Severity (ETDRS) charts. The ETDRS letter score ranges from 0 to 100 (best score)	from baseline to an averaged EDTRS letter score between 24 and 32 weeks and between 48 and 56 weeks
Mean averaged ETDRS letter score	Best Corrected Visual Acuity (BCVA) is measured via Early Treatment Diabetic Retinopathy Severity (ETDRS) charts. The ETDRS letter score ranges from 0 to 100 (best score)	between 24 and 32 weeks and between 48 and 56 weeks

Proportion of eyes gaining ≥5 EDTRS letters		from baseline to an averaged ETDRS letter score between 24 and 32 weeks and between 48 and 56 weeks
Proportion of eyes loosing ≥5 EDTRS letters		from baseline to an averaged ETDRS letter score between 24 and 32 weeks and between 48 and 56 weeks
Mean change in low-luminance Best Corrected Visual Acuity (BCVA)		from baseline to last visit at or before 32 weeks and last visit at or before 56 weeks
Mean change in central subfield thickness (CST)	CST is measured using optical coherence tomography (OCT)	from baseline to an averaged CST between 24 and 32 weeks and between 48 and 56 weeks
Proportion of eyes with no intraretinal fluid	Intraretinal fluid is assessed via optical coherence tomography (OCT)	at baseline, last visit at or before 32 weeks, and at or before 56 weeks
Proportion of eyes with no subretinal fluid	Subretinal fluid is assessed via optical coherence tomography (OCT)	at baseline, last visit at or before 32 weeks, and at or before 56 weeks
Proportion of eyes with no intra- and subretinal fluid	Intra- and subretinal fluid is assessed via optical coherence tomography (OCT)	at baseline, last visit at or before 32 weeks, and at or before 56 weeks
Retinal nerve fiber layer (RNFL) thickness	RNFL thickness is assessed via optical coherence tomography (OCT)	at baseline, last visit at or before 32 weeks, and last visit at or before 56 weeks
Concentration of plasma vascular endothelial growth factor A (VEGF-A) and Angiopoietin-2 (Ang-2)	Plasma VEGF-A and Ang-2 are determined using a validated enzyme-linked immunosorbent assay (ELISA)	at baseline, one week after baseline, four weeks after baseline, and the last visit at or before 32 weeks
Patient-reported vision-related functioning and quality of life	Patient-reported vision-related functioning and quality of life are assessed via the National Eye Institute Visual Function Questionnaire (VFQ-25). VFQ-25 score ranges from 0 to 100 (highest score)	at screening, last visit at or before 32 weeks, and the last visit at or before 56 weeks
Presence of safety outcomes	Rates of adverse events (AE's) and serious adverse events (SAE's) are given	from baseline through to week 56

Sponsor
Medical University of Graz

Collaborators
No information provided

Investigators
- Principal Investigator: Andreas Wedrich, MD, Department of Ophthalmology, Medical University Graz

General Publications
No publications available

Austria

Recruiting

Therapy of Age-Related Macular Degeneration (MET)

ClinicalTrials.gov ID NCT05222997

Sponsor Robert Hörantner
Information provided by Robert Hörantner, Krankenhaus der Barmherzigen Schwestern Ried (Responsible Party)
Last Update Posted 2022-08-18

Study Overview

Brief Summary
People with the disease age-related macular degeneration (AMD) are treated with the Medical Eye Trainer (MET) system to improve their vision. The training is carried out over 2 months.

Detailed Description
Age-related macular degeneration (AMD) is a widespread eye disease worldwide. According to the Gutenberg Health Study, about 7000000 people in Germany suffer from it. The numbers for Austria are to be assumed with 700000 due to the smaller population. There are two different forms of AMD, the wet form with 15% and the dry form with 85%. Both types have a high risk of rapid development of significant visual impairment. For the dry form of the disease, there are currently only a few therapeutic options. The main one is the nutritional supplement therapy. This treatment can only reduce the progression of deterioration in 10% of affected individuals, but there is a significant side effect profile. Thus, the question arose for completely different treatment approaches. For this reason, the Medical Eye Trainer (MET) was developed. This is a training device that can easily be used in self-application. The purpose of this new therapy is not to try to cure AMD. Instead, the eye and brain are trained to better cope with the disease. In the first study on 17 eyes, 11 cases even showed an improvement in visual performance, the remaining 6 cases showed a stable situation. In no case did a deterioration occur. Thus, for the first time, it was possible not only to slow down this disease but even to achieve an improvement. In a second study with a planned number of 150 persons, this positive

effect will be further investigated. A calculation with G*Power, based on the results of the first study, results in an optimal number of 150 examinations.

The participants will be examined in the hospital Ried im Innkreis and treated by MET. No additional measures are required for the study besides the usual eye examinations in AMD.

The study is open to individuals with dry AMD, regardless of age. Exclusion criteria are wet AMD, epilepsy, and double vision. Other eye diseases are not a problem.

The diagnosis is additionally confirmed by an examination of the ocular fundus with an Optical Coherence Tomography (OCT). As an essential factor of the severity of the disease, the visual performance for distance (5–6 m) and for near (40 cm) is determined.

Participants need a mobile electronic device with the operating system Apple IOS® or Android®. The MET training system in the form of software will be provided for the duration of the study. The therapy is performed daily by the patient him/herself and lasts 90 seconds per eye. A success control is planned after two months. The above-mentioned examinations will be repeated.

The MET has a CE approval in the sense of MPG class 1. This study will be performed according to the Helsinki criteria.

Official Title
Therapy of Age-Related Macular Degeneration Through Training with the Medical Eye Trainer

Conditions
Age-Related Macular Degeneration

Intervention/Treatment

Other Study ID Numbers
- 1241/2021

Study Start (Actual)
2022-02-28

Primary Completion (Estimated)
2022-12-31

Study Completion (Estimated)
2023-04-30

Enrollment (Estimated)
150

Study Type
Observational

Austria
Upperaustria Locations

Ried Im Innkreis, Upperaustria, Austria, A—4910
Recruiting
BHS Ried

Contact
Robert Hörantner, MD
00437752602 robert.hoerantner@bhs.at

Contact
Lucie Junger, MD
00437752603 lucie.junger@bhs.at

Eligibility Criteria
Description

Inclusion Criteria
- Age-related macular degeneration

Exclusion Criteria
- Epilepsy
- Double vision
- Study Population
- All persons with dry AMD who have no risk of reacting to the intense visual stimulus with a seizure. Existing double images are intensified by the increased visual acuity. All other affected persons can participate in the training.

Ages Eligible for Study
(Child, Adult, Older Adult)

Sexes Eligible for Study
All

Accepts Healthy Volunteers
No
Sampling Method
Probability Sample

Design Details
Observational Model: Case-Only
Time Perspective: Prospective

Primary outcome measures

Outcome measure	Measure description	Time frame
Change in visual acuity		2 months

Sponsor
Robert Hörantner

Collaborators
No information provided

Investigators
No information provided

General Publications
No publications available

China

Not Yet Recruiting

A Study to Compare LY09004 and Eylea in the Treatment of Wet Age-Related Macular Degeneration (wAMD)

ClinicalTrials.gov ID NCT04572698

Sponsor Luye Pharma Group Ltd.
Information provided by Luye Pharma Group Ltd. (Responsible Party)
Last Update Posted 2020-10-01

Study Overview

Brief Summary
A randomized, double-blind, parallel controlled, multicenter clinical trial to compare the efficacy and safety of LY09004 and EYLEA in the Treatment of Wet Age-related Macular Degeneration (wAMD).

Detailed Description
This is a randomized, double-blind, parallel-controlled, multicenter clinical trial.

The primary objective is to assess the efficacy similarity of LY09004 and EYLEA in the treatment of w-AMD.

The secondary objective is to assess the safety similarity of LY09004 and EYLEA in the treatment of w-AMD.

Official Title
To Compare the Efficacy and Safety of Recombinant Human Vascular Endothelial Growth Factor Receptor Antibody Fusion Protein Eye Injection (LY09004) and Eylea in the Treatment of Wet Age-Related Macular Degeneration (wAMD): A Randomized, Double-Blind, Parallel Controlled, Multicenter Clinical Trial

Conditions
Age-Related Macular Degeneration

Intervention/Treatment
- Drug: LY09004
- Drug: Eylea

Other Study ID Numbers
- LY09004/CT-CHN-302
- Study Start (Estimated)
- 2020-11

Primary Completion (Estimated)
2023-06

Study Completion (Estimated)
2023-12

Enrollment (Estimated)
416

Study Type
Interventional

Phase
Phase 3

Study Contact
Name: Youxin Chen
Phone Number: 8613801025972
Email: chenyouxinpumch@163.com
No location data

Eligibility Criteria
Description

Inclusion Criteria
- The patient or their legal representatives must give the written informed consent form voluntarily
- Aged ≥50 years, male or female
- Patients confirmed diagnosis of w-AMD, currently have active lesions, which are defined as any of the following in the macular area: ① intraretinal fluid; ② intraretinal lipid exudation; ③ subretinal fluid; ④ subretinal hemorrhage; and ⑤ retinal pigment epithelium detachment
- The total area of all types of lesions in the study eye ≤30 mm^2 (the area of 12 optic discs)
- The BCVA between 73 and 24 letters (including boundary values) in the study eye is inclusive using the ETDRS, which is equivalent to 20/40 to 20/320 of Snellen
- Nonstudy eye use ETDRS testing to detect BCVA ≥19 letters, which is equivalent to 20/400 of Snellen
- At the time of screening, childbearing-age (such as women who have not undergone surgical sterilization or have been postmenopausal for less than one year) have a negative blood pregnancy test result. Childbearing-age males and females agree to take effective contraceptive measures throughout the study period and for at least 3 months after medication

Exclusion Criteria

- Any opacity of refractive media or nondilated pupils in the study eye interference with visual acuity detection and the evaluation of anterior segment and fundus
- Study eye retinal hemorrhage ≥4 optic disc area
- Central fovea of the study eye affected by geographic atrophy, scars or fibrosis, dense subfoveal exudation, and macula center affected by retinal pigment epithelium (RPE) tear
- Any concurrent conditions in the study eye that affects central vision (such as diabetic retinopathy, retinal vein occlusion, uveitis, vascular streaks, pathological myopia, retinal detachment, macular hole, epimacular membrane, toxoplasmosis, optic nerve disease, polypoid choroidal vascular disease (PCV), etc.)
- Any history of the following ophthalmic surgery in the study eye: vitrectomy, anti-glaucoma surgery, and macular transposition
- Any evidence of external eye surgery within 1 month or cataract surgery within 3 months before screening in the study eye
- Any the following treatment in the study eye within 3 months before screening: Verteporfin photodynamic therapy (PDT), macular laser photocoagulation, transpupillary thermotherapy (TTT), and other operations for the treatment of AMD
- Aphakia (excluding intraocular lens) or posterior lens capsule rupture (except for YAG laser posterior capsulotomy after intraocular lens implantation more than 1 month from screening) in the study
- Afferent pupil defect (APD) in the study eye
- Patients have received anti-VEGF (vascular endothelial growth factor) treatment within 6 months before screening, such as ranibizumab, bevacizumab, and conbercept in any eye or the whole body
- Use of intraocular or systemic corticosteroids within 3 months before screening or use of periocular corticosteroids within 1 month
- Any active intraocular or periocular infection (for example, blepharitis, infectious conjunctivitis, keratitis) in either eye
- Any history of glaucoma
- Any evidence of pseudocapsular exfoliation syndrome in either eye
- A history of vitreous hemorrhage within 3 months before screening in either eye
- Any systemic drug (currently in use or may need to be used) could cause lens toxicity or retinal toxicity, such as desferrioxamine, chloroquine/hydroxychloroquine, tamoxifen, phenothiazine, and ethambutol
- History of allergy to the therapeutic or diagnostic drugs used in the research protocol, including allergies to the test articles
- Diabetic subjects with diabetic retinopathy or glycosylated hemoglobin>9%
- Any history of surgery within 1 month before screening, and/or any currently unhealed wounds, ulcers, fractures, etc.
- Any infectious disease requiring systemic treatment (oral, intramuscular, or intravenous) during screening
- History of a medical condition, including myocardial infarction, unstable angina pectoris, coronary revascularization, cerebrovascular accidents (including TIA),

other thromboembolic diseases (such as thromboembolic angiitis, pulmonary embolism, deep vein thrombosis, and portal vein thrombosis), New York Heart Association (NYHA) grade ≥ Grade II cardiac insufficiency, severely unstable ventricular arrhythmia within 6 months before screening

- History of diffuse intravascular coagulation and obvious bleeding tendency (such as hemoptysis, hematemesis, and severe purpura) within 3 months before screening, or use of anticoagulant and antiplatelet therapy other than aspirin/NSAIDs within 14 days before screening
- Subjects with systemic immune diseases
- Poorly controlled blood pressure (defined as: after receiving antihypertensive drugs, the subject's systolic value ≥160 mmHg or diastolic value ≥100 mmHg at seat)
- Any uncontrollable clinical disease (such as serious mental, respiratory, and other system diseases and malignant tumors)
- Abnormal liver and kidney function (ALT, AST ≥ 2.5 times the upper limit of normal; total bilirubin≥1.5 times the upper limit of normal; creatinine, urea/urea nitrogen≥1.2 times the upper limit of normal)
- Abnormal blood coagulation function (prothrombin time > upper limit of normal value 3 seconds or activated partial thromboplastin time > upper limit of normal value 10 seconds)
- Positive Hepatitis B surface antigen (HBsAg) and peripheral blood hepatitis B virus deoxyribonucleic acid (HBV DNA) titer test ≥1 × 103 copies/mL; under the condition of positive HBsAg with peripheral blood HBV DNA titer test <1x 10^3 copies/mL, if the investigator judges that chronic hepatitis B is stable and will not increase the risk of the subject, the subject is eligible for selection
- Positive Hepatitis C virus (HCV) antibody, Treponema pallidum antibody, and human immunodeficiency virus (HIV) antibody
- Nursing (lactating) women
- Participation in clinical trials of any drug (excluding vitamins and minerals) within 3 months before screening
- Others need to be excluded according to the judgement of the investigator

Ages Eligible for Study
50 Years and Older (Adult, Older Adult)

Sexes Eligible for Study
All

Accepts Healthy Volunteers
No

Design Details
Primary Purpose: Treatment
Allocation: Randomized
Interventional Model: Parallel Assignment
Masking: Double (Participant Investigator)

Arms and interventions

Participant group/arm	Intervention/treatment
Experimental: LY09004 LY09004 injection by intraocular injection on Day 1, Day 29, Day 57, Day 113, Day 169, Day 225, Day 281 and Day 337	Drug: LY09004 • LY09004 injection by intraocular injection on Day 1, Day 29, Day 57, Day 113, Day 169, Day 225, Day 281, and Day 337 • Other Names: –Recombinant Human Vascular Endothelial Growth Factor Receptor Antibody Fusion Protein Eye Injection
Active Comparator: EYLEA EYLEA injection by intraocular injection on Day 1, Day 29, Day 57, Day 113, Day 169, Day 225, Day 281, and Day 337	Drug: Eylea • EYLEA injection by intraocular injection on Day 1, Day 29, Day 57, Day 113, Day 169, Day 225, Day 281, and Day 337

Primary outcome measures

Outcome measure	Measure description	Time frame
BCVA(best-corrected visual acuity)	Assess the BCVA change similarity from the baseline of LY09004 and EYLEA	week 24

Secondary outcome measures

Outcome measure	Measure description	Time frame
BCVA	Assess the BCVA change similarity from the baseline of LY09004 and EYLEA	week 4, week 8, week 12, week 16, week 20, week 28, week 32, week 36, week 40, week 44, week 48, week 52
Letter	Proportion of subjects with 5/10/15 letters more than baseline in the study eye	week 24, week 52
Central thickness	Changes of central thickness from baseline in study eyes	week 24, week 52
CNV (Choroidal neovascularization) leakage area	Changes of CNV leakage area of study eye compared with baseline	week 24, week 52

Other outcome measures

Outcome measure	Measure description	Time frame
AE (adverse event)	Number of patients with treatment-related adverse events assessed by change from baseline	week 52

Sponsor

Luye Pharma Group Ltd.

Collaborators

- Shan Dong Boan Biotechnology Co., Ltd (Co-sponsor)

Investigators

- Principal Investigator: Youxin Chen, Peking Union Medical College Hospital

General Publications
No publications available

China

Recruiting

Compare the Efficacy and Safety of HLX04-O with Ranibizumab in Subjects with wAMD

ClinicalTrials.gov ID NCT05003245

Sponsor Shanghai Henlius Biotech
Information provided by Shanghai Henlius Biotech (Responsible Party)
Last Update Posted 2022-04-28

Study Overview

Brief Summary
This study will compare the efficacy and safety of HLX04-O administered by IVT with ranibizumab in patients with active CNV secondary to AMD.

Detailed Description
This is a Phase 3, multicenter, randomized double-masked active-controlled study to compare the efficacy and safety of HLX04-O administered by IVT with ranibizumab in patients with active CNV secondary to AMD. The study will be conducted in approximately 60 sites in China.

Either HLX04-O (1.25 mg) IVT or ranibizumab (0.5 mg) IVT will be administered at a 4-week interval for 1 year (12 cycles).

Official Title
A Phase 3 Randomized Double-Masked Active Controlled Study to Compare the Efficacy and Safety of HLX04-O Administered by Intravitreal Injection with Ranibizumab in Subjects with Wet Age-Related Macular Degeneration (wAMD)

Conditions
Age-Related Macular Degeneration

Intervention/Treatment
- Drug: HLX04-O, recombinant anti-vascular endothelial growth factor (VEGF) humanized monoclonal antibody ophthalmic injection
- Drug: Lucentis

Other Study ID Numbers
- HLX04-O-wAMD-CN

Study Start (Actual)
2021-11-01

Primary Completion (Estimated)
2023-08-31

Study Completion (Estimated)
2024-03-31

Enrollment (Estimated)
388

Study Type
Interventional

Phase
Phase 3

Study Contact
Name: Qi Jin, Bachelor
Phone Number: +86-15955160489
Email: qi_jin@henlius.com
China
Anhui Locations

Bengbu, Anhui, China
Recruiting
The first affiliated hospital of Bengbu Medical College

Contact
Wei Wan
0552-3085746 419117369@qq.com

Hefei, Anhui, China
Recruiting
The Second Affiliated Hospital of Anhui Medical University

Contact
Bin Yu
0551-65997421 officegcp@ayefy.com

Beijing Locations

Beijing, Beijing, China
Recruiting
Beijing Tongren Hospital, Capital Medical University

Contact
Yuyang Dai
010-5826848-8001/13811057723 bjtrgcp@163.com

Beijing, Beijing, China
Recruiting
Chinese PLA General Hospital

Contact
Beibei Liang
010-66939409 113910635134@163.com

Beijing, Beijing, China
Recruiting
Xuanwu Hospital, Capital Medical University

Contact
Guanbo Lv
010-63131272 xwgcpht@xwh.ccmu.edu.cn

Chongqing Locations

Chongqing, Chongqing, China
Recruiting
The First Affiliated Hospital of Third Military Medical University (Southwest Hospital)

Contact
Mr Pan
023-68766775 993725117@qq.com

Chongqing, Chongqing, China
Recruiting
The Second Affiliated Hospital of Chongqing Medical University

Contact
Xiaohong Long
023-62888290 chongergcp@163.com

Gansu Locations

Lanzhou, Gansu, China
Recruiting
The Second Hospital of Lanzhou University

Contact
Wen Qiu
0931-8487117 ldeygcp@163.com

Guangdong Locations

Guangzhou, Guangdong, China
Recruiting
The First Affiliated Hospital of Jinan University (Guangzhou Overseas Chinese Hospital)

Contact
Qingcui Huang
020-38688462 drugbase@163.com

Guangzhou, Guangdong, China
Recruiting
Zhujiang Hospital of Southern Medical University

Contact
Rui Li
020-62783374 zjyygcp@163.com

Jieyang, Guangdong, China
Recruiting
Jieyang People's Hospital

Contact
Haowei Liu
0663-8660801 project_jysrmyy@126.com

Guangxi Locations

Nanjing, Guangxi, China
Recruiting
The First Affiliated Hospital of Guangxi Medical University

Contact
Yanwen Zhou
0771- 5356080 gxzywjg@163.com

Nanning, Guangxi, China
Recruiting
The People's Hospital of Guangxi Zhuang Autonomous Region

Contact
Xuemei Huang
0771-2186377 hxm1009@126.com

Guizhou Locations

Guiyang, Guizhou, China
Recruiting
Affiliated Hospital of Guizhou Medical University

Contact
Lin Liu
+86(851)867528172668092677

Zunyi, Guizhou, China
Recruiting
The First People's Hospital of Zunyi

Contact
Yuanyuan Li
0851-23233831 zsyygcp@126.com

Hebei Locations

Cangzhou, Hebei, China
Recruiting
Cangzhou Central Hospital

Contact
Xiaoyang Sun
0317-2072825 czzxyygcp@126.com

Heilongjiang Locations

Ha'erbin, Heilongjiang, China
Recruiting
The First Affiliated Hospital of Harbin Medical University

Contact
Xiaohui Ren
0451-85552399 renxiaohui2004@163.com

Henan Locations

Luoyang, Henan, China
Recruiting
Luoyang Third People's Hospital

Contact
Yan Chen
0379-63963566 lysygcp@163.com

Xinxiang, Henan, China
Recruiting
The First Affiliated Hospital of Xinxiang Medical College

Contact
Chun Liang
0373-4404384 yfygcp4384@163.com

Xinxiang, Henan, China
Recruiting
The Third Affiliated Hospital of Xinxiang Medical College

Contact
Yi Wang
0373-3029575 xysfygcp@163.com

Zhengzhou, Henan, China
Recruiting
Henan Eye Hospital

Contact
Huijuan He
0371-67120925 hehui0111@126.com

Hubei Locations

Wuhan, Hubei, China
Recruiting
People's Hospital of Wuhan University (Hubei Provincial People's Hospital)

Contact
Tiantian Duan
027-88237069 3375565387@qq.com

Wuhan, Hubei, China
Recruiting
Tongji Hospital, Tongji Medical College, Huazhong University of Science and Technology

Contact
Chang Shu
027-83663940 tongjigcp@163.com

Wuhan, Hubei, China
Recruiting
Wuhan AIER Eye Hospital

Contact
Xin Chen
027-68893766 whaiergcp@163.com

Wuhan, Hubei, China
Recruiting
Wuhan Puren Hospital

Contact
Man Lv
027-86360089 Prjgb_gcp@126.com

Yichang, Hubei, China
Recruiting
Yichang Central People's Hospital

Contact
Liling Hu
0717-6487063 ycsgcp@163.com

Jiangxi Locations

Nanchang, Jiangxi, China
Recruiting
Affiliated Eye Hospital of Nanchang University

Contact
Lin Yuan
13803527527 361188958@qq.com

Nanchang, Jiangxi, China
Recruiting
the First Affiliated Hospital of Nanchang University

Contact
Jinhua Wen
0791-88695051 ncuyfygcp2018@163.com

Pingxiang, Jiangxi, China
Recruiting
Pingxiang People's Hospital

Contact
Lv Xiao
0799-6881723 pxsrmyygcp@163.com

Jilin Locations

Jilin, Jilin, China
Recruiting
The First Hospital of Jilin University

Contact
Fei Wang
0431-88786014 wangfei5780@126.com

Liaoning Locations

Shenyang, Liaoning, China
Recruiting
Shenyang AIER Eye Hospital

Contact
Tongshan Zhang
15004008229 tszhang61@163.com

Ningxia Locations

Yinchuan, Ningxia, China
Recruiting
Ningxia Hui Autonomous Region Peoples Hospital

Contact
Xnyuan Cao
0951-5920163

Shandong Locations

Jinan, Shandong, China
Recruiting
Shangdong Provincial Hospital

Contact
Xiaoxuan Huang
0531-68776009 shiyanjigouban@126.com

Qingdao, Shandong, China
Recruiting
The Affiliated Hospital of Qingdao University

Contact
Xin Li
0532-82912263 jidi1767@126.com

Weifang, Shandong, China
Recruiting
Weifang Eye Hospital

Contact
Pengfei Jiang
18363691272 wfykyyjgb@163.com

Shanghai Locations

Shanghai, Shanghai, China, 200233
Recruiting
Shanghai General Hospital

Contact
Xun Xu

Shanghai, Shanghai, China
Recruiting
Shanghai Tenth People's Hospital

Contact
Fei Teng
021-66301632 sygcp2013@126.com

Shanxi Locations

Taiyuan, Shanxi, China
Recruiting
Shanxi Eye Hospital

Contact
Li Wang
13753124052 sxykywjg@163.com

Tianjin Locations

Tianjin, Tianjin, China
Recruiting
Tianjin Eye Hospital

Contact
Yi Zhang
15522516709 tjsykyy@163.com

Zhejiang Locations

Hangzhou, Zhejiang, China
Recruiting
Zhejiang Provincial People's Hospital

Contact
Ying Wang
0571-85893646 zzsrmyygcp@163.c0m

Lishui, Zhejiang, China
Recruiting
Lishui Municioal Central Hospital

Contact
Yayan Zhu
0578-2285718 lsszxyygcp@163.com

Eligibility Criteria
Description

Inclusion Criteria
- Capable of understanding and signing the informed consent form (ICF) which includes compliance with the ICF and this protocol. In the Investigator's judgment, willing and able to complete all visits and assessments adhering to the prohibitions and restrictions specified in this protocol
- Women or men aged ≥50 years when signing the ICF
- Newly diagnosed, untreated, active subfoveal, or juxtafoveal CNV lesions secondary to AMD in the study eye (active CNV was defined as leakage on FA and subretinal or intraretinal fluid on OCT with confirmation of the reading center during screening)
- The total lesion area (including hemorrhage, scar, and neovascularization) of the study eye ≤12 disc area (DA) with confirmation of the reading center before randomization
- The BCVA letters between 24 and 73, inclusive, in the study eye, using Early Treatment Diabetic Retinopathy Study (ETDRS) charts
- Clear ocular media and adequate pupillary dilatation to allow the acquisition of good-quality retinal images to confirm the diagnosis
- Participants' fellow (nonstudy) eye must have had a BCVA of 24 letters or better

Exclusion Criteria

- Macular-related retinal pigment epithelial tears in the study eye; scar, fibrosis, or atrophy involving the fovea, or CNV due to other causes in the study eye (e.g., ocular histoplasmosis, trauma, or pathological myopia) with confirmation of the reading center
- The fellow (nonstudy) eye needs anti-VEGF IVT injection (e.g., CNV due to wAMD, trauma, pathological myopia, retina vein occlusion, diabetic macular edema, etc.) in the next 3 months after randomization, in the investigator's judgment
- Active or recent (within 1 month prior to dose 1) intraocular, extraocular, or periocular infection (including conjunctivitis, keratitis, scleritis, or endophthalmitis), or history of idiopathic or autoimmune-associated uveitis in either eye
- Vitreous hemorrhage in the study eye within 3 months prior to dose 1
- Aphakia (except intraocular lens) or posterior capsular rupture of the lens (except yttrium aluminum-garnet (YAG) laser posterior capsulotomy after intraocular lens implantation ≥1 month prior to first dose) in the study eye
- Corneal dystrophy or history of corneal transplantation, scleral softening or history of scleral softening, history of rhegmatogenous retinal detachment, or macular hole (Stage II, III, or IV) in the study eye
- Uncontrolled glaucoma (defined as intraocular pressure [IOP] ≥25 mmHg despite treatment with antiglaucoma medication) and/or glaucoma filtering surgery (e.g., trabeculectomy, scleral nipping, nonpenetrating trabeculectomy, etc.) or advanced glaucoma resulting in a cup/disc ratio > 0.8 in the study eye
- Equivalent spherical diopter of the study eye ≥-8D. For participants who had undergone refractive correction or cataract surgery, the equivalent spherical diopter of the study eye before surgery ≥-8D
- Estimated by the Investigator, any concurrent intraocular condition except wAMD (e.g., diabetic retinopathy, dry AMD, retina vein occlusion, uveitis, angioid streaks, retinal detachment, epiretinal membrane, amblyopia, central serous chorioretinopathy, etc.) in the study eye that limited the potential to gain visual acuity upon treatment with the investigational product, or could have required medical or surgical intervention during the study to prevent or treat visual loss
- Underwent intraocular surgery including verteporfin photodynamic therapy (PDT), transpupillary thermotherapy, macular translocation, vitrectomy, laser photocoagulation in the macular area, other surgery in the macular area, or surgery to treat AMD
- Previous extraocular or periocular surgery within 1 month or intraocular surgery (including cataract surgery, etc.) within 3 months prior to dose 1, or current unhealed wound, moderate or severe ulcer or history of fracture in the study eye
- Subconjunctival or intraocular or systemic use of corticosteroids within 3 months (including subconjunctival or intraocular long-acting implant within 6 months) prior to dose 1 in the study eye
- Previous systemic anti-VEGF therapy or IVT injection of any anti-VEGF drug into either eye or other ocular use of anti-VEGF drug within 3 months prior to dose 1

- Participated in any drug (other than vitamins and minerals) or device clinical trials within 3 months or the duration of 5 half-lives of the study drug (which is longer) prior to dose 1 and have used the test drug or received device treatment
- Pregnancy or lactation
- Infertile women fail to meet either of the following ones: 1) menopause (≥12 continuous months of amenorrhea with no identified cause other than menopause before screening); 2) surgically sterilized

Men or fertile women fail to meet both of the following ones: 1) women of childbearing potential must have a negative urine or serum pregnancy test result within 14 days prior to the initiation of the study intervention, and should not breastfeed. If the urine pregnancy test is positive, it must be confirmed by a serum pregnancy test; 2) agreement to remain abstinent (refrain from heterosexual intercourse) or use effective contraceptive methods from signed ICF for at least 6 months following the last dose of the study intervention. Effective contraceptive methods include bilateral tubal ligation, male sterilization, established, proper use of hormonal contraceptives that inhibit ovulation, hormone-releasing intrauterine devices (IUDs), and copper IUDs.

- In the Investigator's judgment, there is evidence of a disease or condition that contraindicates the use of an investigational drug or that might affect the interpretation of the results of the study or render the participant at high risk for treatment complications (e.g., stroke or myocardial infarction within 6 months prior todose1, uncontrolled hypertension (systolic blood pressure ≥ 160 mmHg, or diastolic blood pressure ≥ 100 mmHg), etc.)
- Uncontrolled diabetes (defined as HbA1c > 10.0%)
- Alanine aminotransferase (ALT) and/or aspartate aminotransferase (AST) is more than twice the upper limit of normal (ULN), and/or serum creatinine is 1.2 times more than the ULN, and is clinically significant in the opinion of the Investigator
- Abnormal coagulation function (prothrombin time ≥ 3 seconds over ULN, activated partial thromboplastin time ≥ 10 seconds over ULN)
- Active disseminated intravascular coagulation and obvious bleeding tendency within 3 months prior to dose 1
- Evidence of significant uncontrolled concomitant diseases such as cardiovascular diseases, nervous system diseases, respiratory system diseases, urinary system diseases, digestive system diseases, and endocrine diseases
- Current treatment for active systemic infection or history of recurrent serious infections
- Known active or suspected autoimmune diseases, requiring systemic immunosuppressive therapy
- Positive for syphilis screening test or positive for human immunodeficiency virus (HIV) screening test
- Known allergy to any component of the study intervention or history of allergy to fluorescein or indocyanine green, any anesthetics or antimicrobial agents used during the course of the study

- In the Investigator's judgment, other conditions are considered not amenable to this study
- Participant who has been diagnosed with COVID-19 or who has received COVID-19 vaccine within 1 month prior to dose 1

Other protocol-defined inclusion and exclusion criteria may apply.

Ages Eligible for Study
50 Years and Older (Adult, Older Adult)

Sexes Eligible for Study
All

Accepts Healthy Volunteers
No

Design Details
Primary Purpose: Treatment
Allocation: Randomized
Interventional Model: Parallel Assignment
Masking: Double (Participant Investigator)

Arms and interventions

Participant group/arm	Intervention/treatment
Experimental: HLX04-O Biologic recombinant anti-VEGF humanized monoclonal antibody	Drug: HLX04-O, recombinant anti-vascular endothelial growth factor (VEGF) humanized monoclonal antibody ophthalmic injection • 0.05 mL solution at a 4-week interval for intravitreal injection
Active Comparator: Ranibizumab Biologic anti-VEGF recombinant humanized monoclonal antibody fragment	Drug: Lucentis • 0.05 mL solution at a 4-week interval for intravitreal injection

Primary outcome measures

Outcome measure	Measure description	Time frame
Mean change of letters from baseline in best-corrected visual acuity (BCVA) at Week 48.	Detailed Outcome Measures will be defined in the Statistical Analysis Plan	from baseline to week 48

Secondary outcome measures

Outcome measure	Measure description	Time frame
Mean change of letters from baseline in the BCVA over time	Detailed Outcome Measures will be defined in the Statistical Analysis Plan	From baseline to week 48
Proportion of patients gaining at least 15/10/5 letters in the BCVA at Week 12, 24, 36, and 48	Detailed Outcome Measures will be defined in the Statistical Analysis Plan	From baseline to week 48

Mean change from baseline in the total area of CNV and the total area of fluorescein leakage on fluorescein angiography (FA) at Weeks 12, 24, and 48	Detailed Outcome Measures will be defined in the Statistical Analysis Plan	From baseline to week 48
Mean change from baseline in central retina thickness (CRT) on optical coherence tomography (OCT) at Week 12, 24, 36, and 48	Detailed Outcome Measures will be defined in the Statistical Analysis Plan	From baseline to week 48
Change from baseline in National Eye Institute Visual Functioning Questionnaire—25 scale score at Weeks 12, 24, and 48	Detailed Outcome Measures will be defined in the Statistical Analysis Plan	From baseline to week 48
Percentage and severity of ocular AEs (IVT procedure-related and Investigation Medication related), nonocular AEs; laboratory abnormalities; vital sign, physical examination abnormalities, etc.	Detailed Outcome Measures will be defined in the Statistical Analysis Plan	From baseline to week 48
Incidence of ADAs and NAbs against HLX04-O following IVT administration	Detailed Outcome Measures will be defined in the Statistical Analysis Plan	From baseline to week 48
HLX04-O serum concentrations before Dose 1, Dose 2, Dose 6, Dose 9, and Dose 12 and the last visit as data permit	Detailed Outcome Measures will be defined in the Statistical Analysis Plan	From baseline to week 48

Sponsor
Shanghai Henlius Biotech

Collaborators
No information provided

Investigators
No information provided

General Publications
No publications available

China

Recruiting

A Phase 3 Study to Compare the Efficacy and Safety of HLX04-O with Ranibizumab in Subjects with wAMD

ClinicalTrials.gov ID NCT04740671

Sponsor Shanghai Henlius Biotech
Information provided by Shanghai Henlius Biotech (Responsible Party)
Last Update Posted 2023-08-31

Study Overview

Brief Summary
This study will compare the efficacy and safety of HLX04-O administered by intravitreal injection (IVT) with ranibizumab in patients with active wAMD.

Detailed Description
This is a Phase 3, Randomized, Double-masked, Active-Controlled Study to Compare the Efficacy and Safety of HLX04-O Administered by Intravitreal Injection with Ranibizumab in Subjects with wet Age-related Macular Degeneration (wAMD). This study will be conducted in approximately 90 sites in different countries or regions.

Official Title
A Phase 3, Randomized, Double-Masked, Active Controlled Study to Compare the Efficacy and Safety of HLX04-O Administered by Intravitreal Injection with Ranibizumab in Subjects with Wet Age-related Macular Degeneration (wAMD)

Conditions
Age-Related Macular Degeneration

Intervention/Treatment
- Drug: HLX04-O
- Drug: ranibizumab

Other Study ID Numbers
- HLX04-O-wAMD

Study Start (Actual)
2021-07-01

Primary Completion (Estimated)
2024-08-30

Study Completion (Estimated)
2024-11-30

Enrollment (Estimated)
388

Study Type
Interventional

Phase
Phase 3

United States
Arizona Locations

Gilbert, Arizona, United States, 85297
Recruiting
Associated Retina Consultants-Gilbert

Contact
Stephen DeSouza
480-999-5458 stephendesouza@yahoo.com

Phoenix, Arizona, United States, 85020
Recruiting
Associated Retina Consultants-Phoenix

Contact
Jaime Gaitan
480-999-5458 jrgaitan@cox.net

California Locations

Huntington Beach, California, United States, 92647
Not yet recruiting
VMR Institute

Contact
J Sebag
714-901-7777 JSebag@vmrinstitute.com

Long Beach, California, United States, 90807
Not yet recruiting
South Coast Retina Center

Contact
Randall Nguyen
562-984-7024 ext 6randallnguyen@yahoo.com

Los Alamitos, California, United States, 90720
Not yet recruiting
Retina Consultants of Orange County

Contact
Adrean Sean
714-738-4620 seadrean@yahoo.com

Los Angeles, California, United States, 90048
Not yet recruiting
MACRO Trials/Lazar Retina

Contact
David Benjamin Lazar
747-288-6530 dblazar@gmail.com

Colorado Locations

Colorado Springs, Colorado, United States, 80909
Recruiting
Retina Consultants of Southern Colorado

Contact
Adam Martidis
719-473-9595 researchmdmartidis@coloradoretina.com

Florida Locations

Fort Lauderdale, Florida, United States, 33309
Not yet recruiting
Pinnacle Research Institute

Contact
Sunir Joshi
954-597-6445 sunirjoshi@gmail.com

Jacksonville, Florida, United States, 32216
Recruiting
Florida Retina Institute-Orlando

Contact
Benjamin Thomas
909-831-3589 bthomas@floridaretinainstitute.com

Orlando, Florida, United States, 32806
Recruiting
Florida Retina Institute-Orlando

Contact
Matthew Cunningham
407-849-9621 macunning@gmail.com

Tampa, Florida, United States, 33612
Not yet recruiting
University of South Florida

Contact
Mamta Patel
813-974-0948 mamtapatel@usf.edu

West Palm Beach, Florida, United States, 33409
Not yet recruiting
Mittleman Eye Center

Contact
Scott Fair
561-500-3937 sfair@mittlemaneye.com

Georgia Locations

Augusta, Georgia, United States, 30909
Recruiting
Southeast Retina Center

Contact
Thomas Marcus
706-650-0061 dmarcus@southeastretina.com

Illinois Locations

Chicago, Illinois, United States, 60637
Not yet recruiting
The University of Chicago, IL

Contact
Skondra Dimitra
217-503-9291 dskondra@bsd.uchicago.edu

Kansas Locations

Lenexa, Kansas, United States, 66215
Recruiting
Retina Associates LLC

Contact
Ivan Batlle
913-601-3562 ivankb@kcretina.com

Minnesota Locations

Edina, Minnesota, United States, 55435
Recruiting
Retina Consultants of Minnesota

Contact
Peter Tang
763-550-1002 peter.h.tang@gmail.com

Minneapolis, Minnesota, United States, 55455
Not yet recruiting
University of Minnesota

Contact
Dara Koozkenani
612-625-4108 dkoozeka@umn.edu

Saint Louis Park, Minnesota, United States, 55416
Recruiting
VitreoRetinal Surgery PLLC DBA Retina Consultants of Minnesota

Contact
Jacob Jones
763-550-1002 drjones@retinamn.com

North Carolina Locations

Wake Forest, North Carolina, United States, 27332
Recruiting
North Carolina Retina Associates

Contact
John Thordsen
919-782-8038 jthordsen@ncretina.com

South Carolina Locations

Beaufort, South Carolina, United States, 29902
Recruiting
Retina Consultants of Charleston—Beaufort

Contact
Jablon Eric
843-763-4466 ext 1404 eric.jablon@retinacharleston.com

Florence, South Carolina, United States, 29501
Not yet recruiting
Carolina Center for Sight

Contact
Rishi Singhal
706-955-6487 rsinghal@ccfs2020.com

Texas Locations

Bellaire, Texas, United States, 77401
Recruiting
Retina Consultants of Texas—Newcastle

Contact
David Brown
713-524-3434 ext 4885 dmbmd@retinaconsultantstexas.com

Houston, Texas, United States, 77015
Not yet recruiting
Mt. Olympus Research-Garcia

Contact
Chales Garcia
832-805-1197 erg.garibay@gmail.com

Houston, Texas, United States, 77074
Not yet recruiting
Clinical Trial Network

Contact
Richard Yee
713-484-6947 fdayani@ctntexas.com

Round Rock, Texas, United States, 78681
Recruiting
Retina Consultants of Texas—Round Rock

Contact
Edward Wood
512-687-7281 ewood@austinretina.com

Sugar Land, Texas, United States, 77479
Not yet recruiting
Mt. Olympus Research-Kavoussi

Contact
Shawn Kavoussi
832-805-1197 drkavoussi@gmail.com

The Woodlands, Texas, United States, 77384
Recruiting
Retina Consultants of Texas

Contact
Charles Wykoff
713-524-3434 ccwmd@retinaconsultantstexas.com

Utah Locations

Salt Lake City, Utah, United States, 84107
Recruiting
Rocky Mountain Retina Consultants

Contact
Mitchell Goff
801-264-4444 mmmgoff@yahoo.com

Australia

Melbourne, Australia
Terminated
The Alfred Hospital

Nedlands, Australia
Recruiting
Lions Eye Institute

Contact
CHANDRAKUMAR BALARATNASINGAM
+61 8 9381 0829 chandra@lei.org.au

Western Australia Locations

Nedlands, Western Australia, Australia, WA 6009
Recruiting
Lions Eye Institute

Contact
Chandrakumar Balaratnasingam, doctor
61 8 6382 0582 balaratnasingam@gmail.com

Bulgaria

Burgas, Bulgaria
Not yet recruiting
Specialized Eye Hospital For Active Treatment—Burgas Ltd

Contact
NIKOLAY IVANOV
359896777165

Montana, Bulgaria
Terminated
Mhat Dr. Stamen Iliev Ad

Plovdiv, Bulgaria
Recruiting
Assoc. Prof. Dr. Desislava Koleva Aipsmaed Sveti Luka Eood

Contact
GEORGIEVA DESISLAVA KOLEVA
+359 876 130 135 dr_desikoleva@yahoo.com

Plovdiv, Bulgaria
Not yet recruiting
Medical Center Dar Plovdiv Ltd

Contact
ANDREY BAKARDZHIEV
359899605655

Sofia, Bulgaria
Recruiting
Dcc Aleksandrovska Eood

Contact
ALEXANDER OSCAR
+359 898 747 258 alekoscar@me.com

Sofia, Bulgaria
Recruiting
Umhat Lozenets Ead

Contact
DIDA KAZAKOVA
+359 889 707 134 dida_kazakova@hotmail.com

Sofia, Bulgaria
Recruiting
University First Mhat—Sofia Sv. Joan Krastitel Ead

Contact
DIMITROV TSVETOMIR
+359 888 702 405 prof.ts.dimitrov@abv.bg

Stara Zagora, Bulgaria
Not yet recruiting
Medical Center Vereya Ltd

Contact
DIMITAR DZHELEBOV
359 888 393 210

Varna, Bulgaria
Recruiting
Specialized Hospital For Active Treatment in Ophthalmology—Varna

Contact
DIMITAR GRUPCHEV
+ 359 897 433 923 dgrupchev@gmail.com

Veliko Tarnovo Locations

Gorna Oryahovitsa, Veliko Tarnovo, Bulgaria
Recruiting
Vizus Eood

Contact
PETYA TSVETANOVA
+359 888 266 935 vizus_bg@abv.bg

China
Gansu Locations

Lanzhou, Gansu, China
Recruiting
Lanzhou University Second Hospital

Contact
Wenfang Zhang
13893205506 zhwenf888@163.com

Guangdong Locations

Shantou, Guangdong, China
Recruiting
Joint Shantou International Eye Center Of Shantou University and the Chinese University of Hong Kong

Contact
Mingzhi Zhang
13829668096 zmz@jsiec.org

Henan Locations

Xinxiang, Henan, China
Recruiting
The Third Affiliated Hospital of Xinxiang Medical University

Contact
Xiangling Liu
13782512332 13782512332@163.com

Jilin Locations

Changchun, Jilin, China
Recruiting
First Hospital of Jilin University

Contact
Jilong Hao
13756661327 haojl@jlu.edu.cn

Ningxia Locations

Yinchuan, Ningxia, China
Recruiting
The People's Hospital of Ningxia Hui Autonomous Region

Contact
Wenjuan Zhuang
13995315885 zh_wenj@163.com

Shandong Locations

Weifang, Shandong, China
Recruiting
Weifang Eye Hospital

Contact
Xinyan Xu
13515366033 76469587@qq.com

Shanghai Locations

Shanghai, Shanghai, China
Recruiting
Shanghai First Peoples' Hospital

Contact
Xun Xu
13386259538 drxuxun@tom.com

Shanxi Locations

Taiyuan, Shanxi, China
Recruiting
Shanxi Eye Hospital

Contact
Dongping Zheng
13934047161 mali02120212@163.com

Czechia

Pardubice, Czechia
Terminated
Oftex Ocni Klinika

Prague, Czechia
Withdrawn
Axon Clinical

Prague, Czechia
Withdrawn
Vseobecna Fakultni Nemocnice V Praze

France

Amiens, France
Terminated
Centre Hospitalier Universitaire Amiens-Picardie Service D'Ophthalmologie Amiens France

Paris, France
Terminated
University Eye Clinic Centre Hospitalier Creteil Paris France

Germany

Bonn, Germany
Recruiting
Ukb University of Bonn

Contact
RAFFAEL LIEGL
4922828719784 raffael.liegl@ukbonn.de

Freiburg, Germany
Recruiting
University Hospital Freiburg

Contact
HANSJURGEN AGOSTINI
4976127040060 hansjuergen.agostini@uniklinik-freiburg.de

Giessen, Germany
Terminated
Justus Liebig University Giessen

Mainz, Germany
Recruiting
Johannes Gutenberg University Mainz

Contact
KATRIN LORENZ
496131174069 katrin.lorenz@unimedizin-mainz.de

Munster, Germany
Recruiting
St Franziskus Hospital Munster

Contact
MATTHIAS GUTFLEISCH
492519352702 matthias.gutfleisch@augen-franziskus.de

Sulzbach, Germany
Terminated
Eye Clinic Sulzbach

Hungary

Budapest, Hungary
Recruiting
Bajcsy-Zsilinszky Korhaz Es Rendelointezet

Contact
AGNES KERENYI
0.999999977 agneskerenyi@gmail.com

Budapest, Hungary
Recruiting
Semmelweis Egyetem

Contact
ANDRAS PAPP
36302410960 andras.papp.md@gmail.com

Eger, Hungary
Recruiting
Markhot Ferenc Oktatokorhaz Es Rendelointezet

Contact
AKOS VADNAY
36 20 422 0708 vadnayszemeszet@gmail.com

Pecs, Hungary
Recruiting
Pecsi Tudomanyegyetem Klinikai Kozpont—Szemeszeti Klinika

Contact
ADRIENNE CSUTAK
36305358975 csutak.adrienne@pte.hu

Pécs, Hungary
Recruiting
Ganglion Orvosi Kozpont

Contact
BALAZS VARSANYI
+3672951130 varsanyi.balazs@gmail.com

Szeged, Hungary
Recruiting
Szegedi Tudomanyegyetem Aok Szakk

Contact
EDIT TOTH-MOLNAR
3662545487 tme@tmedit.hu

Italy

Milan, Italy
Terminated
Clinica Oculistica Ospedale Luigi Sacco, Universita' Degli Studi Di Milano

Milan, Italy
Terminated
Clinica Oculistica Universita Vita Salute—Irccs Ospedale San Raffaele

Rome, Italy
Terminated
Fondazione Policlinico Universitario Agostino Gemelli—Irccs Uoc Oculistica

Rome, Italy
Terminated
Irccs Fondazione G.B. Bietti Per Lo Studio E La Ricerca in Oftalmologia Onlus
Rome, Italy

Latvia

Riga, Latvia
Recruiting
P Stradina Clinical University Hospital

Contact
GUNA LAGANOVSKA
37129106879 glaganovska@ml.lv

Riga, Latvia
Recruiting
Riga East University Hospital

Contact
KRISTINE BAUMANE
37126520449 baumanek@ml.lv

Poland

Bydgoszcz, Poland
Recruiting
Oftalmika Sp Z.O.O

Contact
BARTLOMIEJ KALUZNY
48533901100 bartka@by.onet.pl

Katowice, Poland
Recruiting
Centrum Klinicke Oftalmologie S.R.O

Contact
Ewa Mrukwa-Kominek
48323581460 mrukwa@uck.katowice.pl

Kraków, Poland
Recruiting
Szpital SW. Rozy

Contact
MALGORZATA SIEWIERSKA
48126371645 tsiewi@wp.pl

Lublin, Poland
Recruiting
Samodzielny Publiczny Szpital Kliniczny Nr 1 W Lubline

Contact
Anna Swiech
48815340251 anna.zub@umlub.pl

Poznan, Poland
Terminated
Szpital SW Wojciecha

Tarnowskie Góry, Poland
Recruiting
Caminomed Wojciech Jedrzejewski

Contact
Wojciech Jedrzejewski
48881343481 caminomed.jedrzejewski@gmail.com

Tarnów, Poland
Recruiting
Centrum Medyczne Uno-Med

Contact
Piotr Oleksy
48146925440 piotroleksy@yahoo.pl

Walbrzych, Poland
Recruiting
Centrum Medyczne Piasta 47

Contact
Ewa Fluder
48505160995 efluder@globebadania.pl

Warsaw, Poland
Terminated
Nzoz Optimed

Warszawa, Poland
Terminated
Retina Okulistyka Sp.Z O.O.Sp.K.

Podlaskie Locations

Bialystok, Podlaskie, Poland
Recruiting
Nzoz E-Vita

Contact
Maciej Walkowiak
48857460986 maciej.walkowiak.evita@gmail.com

WA Locations

Krakow, WA, Poland
Recruiting
Centrum Medyczne Promed

Contact
Michal Orski
48124151101 orski.michal@gmail.com

Serbia

Belgrade, Serbia
Recruiting
Special Optalmological Hospital Belgrade

Contact
Marko Kontic
381641290623 markokontic@gmail.com

Belgrade, Serbia
Recruiting
Zvezdara University Medical Center

Contact
Miroslav Stamenkovic
381641180115 drmiroslavstamenkovic@gmail.com

Singapore

Singapore, Singapore
Terminated
National University Hospital

Slovakia

Banská Bystrica, Slovakia
Recruiting
Ocna Klinika Szu F.D.R.Banska Bystrica

Contact
Ladislav Janco
4210484412147 ljanco@nspbb.sk

Nitra, Slovakia
Recruiting
Fakultna Nemocnica Nitra

Contact
Gabriela Pavlovicova
421 356 912 503 gabriela.pavlovicova@fnnitra.sk

Nové Zámky, Slovakia
Recruiting
Fakultna Nemocnica S Poliklinikou Nove Zamky Oftalmologicke Nelozkove Oddelenie

Contact
LUBICA BRANIKOVA
421356912503 lubica.branikova@nspnz.sk

Poprad, Slovakia
Recruiting
Nemocnica Poprad As Oftalmologicke Oddelenie Jzs

Contact
LIVIA JAVORSKA
+42152712542 petra.senesiova@gmail.com

Trebišov, Slovakia
Recruiting
Nemocnica S Poliklinikou Trebisov A.S. Ocne Oddelenie Jzs

Contact
MARIA HURCIKOVA
+4210566722443 maria.hurcikova@svetzdravia.com

Trenčianske Teplice, Slovakia
Recruiting
Fakultna Nemocnica Trencin

Contact
MAREK KACERIK
+421 (0) 32-6566-388 marek.kacerik@fntn.sk

Žilina, Slovakia
Recruiting
Fakultna Nemocnica S Poliklinikou Zilina

Contact
MIKULAS ALEXIK
+421 041 5110 366 mikulas.alexik@gmail.com

Spain

Alicante, Spain
Recruiting
VISSUM

Contact
PEDRO AMAT
34965154062 pedroamat@vissum.com

Barcelona, Spain
Recruiting
Centro de Oftalmologia Barraquer

Contact
SANTIAGO ABENGOECHEA HERNANDEZ
34932095311 sah@barraquer.com

Barcelona, Spain
Recruiting
Hospital Universitari Vall D Hebron

Contact
MIGUEL ANGEL ZAPATA VICTORI
34655809682 mazapata@vhebron.net

Barcelona, Spain
Recruiting
Instítito de Microcirugia Ocular

Contact
CECILIA SALINAS
34932531500 salinas@imo.es

Barcelona, Spain
Recruiting
Institut Catala de La Retina

Contact
IGNASI JURGENS MESTRE
34933782319 jurgens@comb.cat

Burjassot, Spain
Recruiting
Oftalvist Clinic

Contact
ROBERTO GALLEGO-PINAZO
+34963003003 robertogallegopinazo@gmail.com

Cordoba, Spain
Recruiting
Hospital La Arruzafa

Contact
JUAN MANUEL CUBERO
+3434957401040 jmcubero@hospitalarruzafa.com

Cordoba, Spain
Withdrawn
Hospital Universitario Reina Sofia

Madrid, Spain
Recruiting
Hospital Clinico San Carlos

Contact
JUAN DONATE LOPEZ
+34913303000x2721 juan.donate@amqoftalmos.es

Madrid, Spain
Terminated
Hospital Universitario Fundacion Jimenez Diaz

Majadahonda, Spain
Recruiting
Hospital Universitario Puerta de Hierro

Contact
JOSE MARIA RUIZ MORENO
34911916000 josemaria.ruiz@uclm.es

Oviedo, Spain
Recruiting
Instituto Oftalmologico Fernandez-Vega

Contact
ALVARO FERNANDEZ-VEGA SANZ
34985240141 sararols.laura@hotmail.com

Pamplona, Spain
Recruiting
Clinica Universitario de Navarra

Contact
ALFERDO GARCIA LAYANA
+34948296 aglayana@unav.es

San Sebastián, Spain
Terminated
Hospital Universitario Donostia

Sant Cugat Del Valles, Spain
Terminated
Omiq Hospital General de Catalunya

Sevilla, Spain
Recruiting
Hospital Universitario Virgen Macarena

Contact
ESTANISLAO GUTIERREZ SANCHEZ
34696402436 esgusan@hotmail.com

Valencia, Spain
Recruiting
Clinica Oftalmologica Aiken

Contact
PATRICIA UDAONDO
34960046566 luisariasbarquet@gmail.com

Valencia, Spain
Recruiting
Consorcio Hospital General Universitario de Valencia

Contact
ENRIQUE CERVERA TAULET
+34963131800x437600 enriquecerverataulet@gmail.com

Valencia, Spain
Recruiting
Fisabio Oftalmologia Medica

Contact
MARIA DEL CARMEN DESCO ESTEBAN
34962787620 carmen.desco@uv.es

Valladolid, Spain
Recruiting
Hospital Rio Hortega

Contact
JAVIER ANTONIO MONTERO MORENO
34630005894 javiermonmor@gmail.com

Zaragoza, Spain
Recruiting
Hospital Universitario Miguel Servet

Contact
LUIS EMILIO PABLO JULVEZ
+34976765500x141089 lpablo@unizar.es

Eligibility Criteria
Description

Inclusion Criteria

- Capable of understanding and signing the informed consent form (ICF) which includes compliance with the requirements and restrictions listed in the ICF and in this protocol
- Women or men aged ≥50 years when signing the ICF
- In the Investigator's judgment, willing and able to complete all visits and assessments adhering to the prohibitions and restrictions specified in this protocol
- Newly diagnosed, untreated, active CNV lesions secondary to age-related macular degeneration that affect the central subfield (CSF) in the study eye. Active CNV was defined as leakage on fluorescein angiography (FA) and subretinal or intraretinal fluid on optical coherence tomography (OCT) with confirmation of the reading center during screening
- The total lesion area (including hemorrhage, scar, and neovascularization) of the study eye ≤12 disc area (DA) with confirmation of the reading center before randomization
- The BCVA letters between 24 and 73, inclusive, in the study eye, using Early Treatment Diabetic Retinopathy Study (ETDRS) charts
- Participants' fellow (nonstudy) eye must have a BCVA of 24 letters or better
- Clear ocular media and adequate pupillary dilatation to allow the acquisition of good-quality retinal images to confirm the diagnosis

Exclusion Criteria

- Macular-related retinal pigment epithelial tears in the study eye; scar, fibrosis, or atrophy involving the fovea, or CNV due to other causes in the study eye (e.g., ocular histoplasmosis, trauma, pathological myopia, etc.) with confirmation of the reading center
- The fellow (nonstudy) eye needs anti-VEGF IVT injection (e.g., CNV due to wAMD, trauma, pathological myopia, retina vein occlusion, diabetic macular edema, etc.) in the next 3 months after randomization, in the investigator's judgment
- Aphakia (except intraocular lens) or posterior capsular rupture of the lens (except yttrium-aluminum-garnet (YAG) laser posterior capsulotomy after intraocular lens implantation ≥30 days prior to first dose) in the study eye
- Active or recent (within 1 month prior to dose 1) intraocular, extraocular, or periocular infection (including conjunctivitis, keratitis, scleritis, or endophthalmitis), or history of idiopathic or autoimmune-associated uveitis in either eye
- Vitreous hemorrhage in the study eye within 3 months prior to dose 1
- Corneal dystrophy or history of corneal transplantation, scleral softening or history of scleral softening, history of rhegmatogenous retinal detachment, or macular hole (Stage II, III, or IV) in the study eye
- Uncontrolled glaucoma in the study eye (defined as intraocular pressure [IOP] ≥25 mmHg despite treatment with antiglaucoma medication) and/or glaucoma

filtering surgery (e.g., trabeculectomy, scleral nipping, nonpenetrating trabeculectomy, etc.)

- Equivalent spherical diopter of the study eye ≥-8D. For participants who had undergone refractive correction or cataract surgery, the equivalent spherical diopter of the study eye before surgery ≥-8D
- Estimated by the Investigator, any concurrent intraocular condition except wAMD (e.g., diabetic retinopathy, dry AMD, retina vein occlusion, uveitis, angioid streaks, retinal detachment, epiretinal membrane, amblyopia, central serous chorioretinopathy, etc.) in the study eye that limited the potential to gain visual acuity upon treatment with the investigational product, or could have required medical or surgical intervention during the study to prevent or treat visual loss
- Underwent intraocular surgery including verteporfin photodynamic therapy (PDT), transpupillary thermotherapy, macular translocation, vitrectomy, laser photocoagulation in the macular area, other surgery in the macular area, or surgery to treat AMD
- Previous extraocular or periocular surgery within 1 month or intraocular surgery (except the surgery mentioned in exclusion 10, such as cataract surgery) within 3 months prior to dose 1, or current unhealed wound, moderate or severe ulcer or fracture in the study eye
- Subconjunctival or intraocular use of corticosteroids within 3 months (including subconjunctival or intraocular long-acting implant within 6 months) prior to dose 1 in the study eye. Use of systemic corticosteroids for 30 or more consecutive days within 3 months prior to dose 1. Inhaled, nasal or dermal steroids are permitted. Topical ocular corticosteroids administered for 30 or more consecutive days in the study eye within 3 months prior to dose 1
- Previous systemic anti-VEGF therapy or IVT injection of any anti-VEGF drug into either eye or other ocular use of anti-VEGF drug within 3 months prior to dose 1
- Participated in any drug (other than vitamins and minerals) or device clinical trials 3 months or the duration of 5 half-lives of the study drug (which is longer) before the first dose and have used the test drug or received device treatment
- Pregnancy or lactation, or fertile men or women not willing to use effective contraception from the day when ICF was signed to at least 6 months following the last dose of study intervention
- Infertile women or men fail to meet either of the following ones: 1) menopause (≥12 continuous months of amenorrhea with no identified cause other than menopause before screening) and 2) surgically sterilized

Fertile women or men fail to meet either of the following ones: (1) women of childbearing potential must have a negative urine or serum pregnancy test result within 14 days prior to initiation of the study intervention, and should not breastfeed. If the urine pregnancy test is positive, it must be confirmed by a serum pregnancy test; (2) agreement to remain abstinent (refrain from heterosexual intercourse) or use effective contraceptive methods from signed ICF for at least 6 months following the last dose of study intervention. Effective contraceptive methods with a failure rate of

<1% per year, including bilateral tubal ligation, male sterilization, established, proper use of hormonal contraceptives that inhibit ovulation, hormone-releasing intrauterine devices (IUDs), and copper IUDs.

- In the Investigator's judgment, there is evidence of a disease or condition that contraindicates the use of an investigational drug or that might affect the interpretation of the results of the study or render the participant at high risk for treatment complications (e.g., stroke or myocardial infarction within 6 months prior to dose 1, uncontrolled hypertension (systolic blood pressure $\geq$ 160 mmHg, or diastolic blood pressure $\geq$ 100 mmHg), etc.)
- Uncontrolled diabetes (defined as HbA1c > 10.0%)
- Alanine aminotransferase (ALT) and/or aspartate aminotransferase (AST) is more than twice the upper limit of normal (ULN), and/or serum creatinine is 1.2 times more than the ULN and is clinically significant in the opinion of the Investigator
- Abnormal coagulation function: prothrombin time (PT) or International normalized ratio (INR) $\geq 1.5 \times$ ULN, or activated partial thromboplastin time (aPTT) $\geq 1.5 \times$ ULN, and is clinically significant in the opinion of the Investigator
- Active disseminated intravascular coagulation and obvious bleeding tendency within 3 months prior to dose 1
- Evidence of significant uncontrolled concomitant diseases such as cardiovascular diseases, nervous system diseases, respiratory system diseases, urinary system diseases, digestive system diseases, and endocrine diseases (e.g., stroke, myocardial infarction)
- Current treatment for active systemic infection or history of recurrent serious infections
- Known active or suspected autoimmune diseases, requiring systemic immunosuppressive therapy
- Positive for syphilis screening test human immunodeficiency virus (HIV) infection or positive for HIV screening test
- Known allergy to any component of the study intervention or history of allergy to fluorescein or indocyanine green, any anesthetics or antimicrobial agents used during the course of the study
- In the Investigator's judgment, other conditions are considered not amenable to this study
- Participant who has been diagnosed with COVID-19 within 2 weeks prior to the first dose, or still symptomatic from an earlier infection (except symptoms associated with "Long COVID "), or displaying symptoms consistent with COVID-19 in the absence of a confirmed COVID-19 infection

Ages Eligible for Study
50 Years and Older (Adult, Older Adult)

Sexes Eligible for Study
All

Accepts Healthy Volunteers
No

Design Details

Primary Purpose: Treatment
Allocation: Randomized
Interventional Model: Parallel Assignment
Masking: Double (Participant Investigator)

Arms and interventions

Participant group/arm	Intervention/treatment
Experimental: HLX04-O Biologic recombinant anti-VEGF humanized monoclonal antibody	Drug: HLX04-O • Biologic recombinant anti-VEGF humanized monoclonal antibody, developed by Shanghai Henlius Biotech, Inc.
Active Comparator: Ranibizumab Biologic anti-VEGF recombinant humanized monoclonal antibody fragment	Drug: ranibizumab • Biologic anti-VEGF recombinant humanized monoclonal antibody fragment

Primary outcome measures

Outcome measure	Measure description	Time frame
Mean change from baseline in BCVA at Week 36	Detailed Outcome Measures will be defined in the Statistical Analysis Plan	up to Week 36

Secondary outcome measures

Outcome measure	Measure description	Time frame
Key Secondary Outcome: Mean change from baseline in BCVA at Week 4.	Detailed Outcome Measures will be defined in the Statistical Analysis Plan	up to Week 48
Mean change in BCVA over time	Detailed Outcome Measures will be defined in the Statistical Analysis Plan	up to Week 48
Proportion of patients gaining at least 15 letters in the BCVA at Weeks 12, 24, 36, and 48	Detailed Outcome Measures will be defined in the Statistical Analysis Plan	up to Weeks 12, 24, 36, and 48
Proportion of patients gaining at least 10 letters in the BCVA at Week 12, 24, 36, and 48	Detailed Outcome Measures will be defined in the Statistical Analysis Plan	up to Weeks 12, 24, 36 and 48
Proportion of patients gaining at least 5 letters in the BCVA at Week 12, 24, 36, and 48	Detailed Outcome Measures will be defined in the Statistical Analysis Plan	up to Weeks 12, 24, 36, and 48
• Mean change from baseline in size of CNV and total area of fluorescein leakage from CNV on FA at Weeks 12, 36, and 48 (as measured by the Reading Center)	Detailed Outcome Measures will be defined in the Statistical Analysis Plan	up to Weeks 12, 36, and 48
• Mean change from baseline in CRT on OCT at Weeks 12, 24, 36, and 48 (as measured by the Reading Center)	Detailed Outcome Measures will be defined in the Statistical Analysis Plan	up to weeks 12, 24, 36, and 48
Change from baseline in NEI VFQ-25 scale score at Weeks 12, 36, and 48	Detailed Outcome Measures will be defined in the Statistical Analysis Plan	up to Weeks 12, 36, and 48

Sponsor
Shanghai Henlius Biotech

Collaborators
No information provided

Investigators
No information provided

General Publications
No publications available

China

Recruiting

Treatment of Recalcitrant Neovascular AMD Using Brolocizumab with Immediate T&E

ClinicalTrials.gov ID NCT05710471

Sponsor The University of Hong Kong
Information provided by Dr. Nicholas Fung, The University of Hong Kong (Responsible Party)
Last Update Posted 2023-02-09

Study Overview

Brief Summary
The investigator proposes to conduct a randomized clinical trial, investigating the safety and efficacy of brolucizumab for the treatment of nAMD patients with CNV, and plans to specifically target those who are not responding to the standard Treat and Extend (T&E) treatment. A randomized study will be conducted with 2 arms, one with the new drug (brolocizumab) and novel treatment protocol versus a second arm using the current gold standard of aflibercept and the T&E protocol.

Detailed Description
In addition, there will also be a rescue option for those in the aflibercept arm who are not responding well to also switch to brolucizumab. The primary outcome is the change in central macular thickness since we expect the new treatment to be effective in reducing intraretinal and subretinal fluids, which in effect are indicators of disease activity. In addition, investigator will look at the improvement of visual acuity, the reduction of treatment intervals, total number of injections over 1 year, recurrence rate, and safety profiles of both drugs.

Official Title
Treatment of Recalcitrant Neovascular AMD Using Brolocizumab with a Novel Treat and Extend Protocol—a Randomized Controlled Prospective Study

Conditions
Age-Related Macular Degeneration

Intervention/Treatment
- Drug: Brolucizumab
- Drug: Aflibercept

Other Study ID Numbers
- Switch Study

Study Start (Actual)
2022-07-25

Primary Completion (Estimated)
2023-07-25

Study Completion (Estimated)
2023-08-30

Enrollment (Estimated)
64

Study Type
Interventional

Phase
Phase 4

Study Contact
Name: Nicholas Fung
Phone Number: 852 39621405
Email: nfung@hku.hk

Study Contact Backup
Name: Ella Lee
Email: eyhlee@hku.hk
Hong Kong

Hong Kong, Hong Kong
Recruiting
Grantham Hospital

Contact
Ella Lee
eyhlee@hku.hk

Eligibility Criteria
Description

Inclusion Criteria
- Age 50 and above
- Diagnosis of exudative age-related macular degeneration (subfoveal CNV) as shown on optical coherence tomography (OCT)—the presence of intraretinal fluid, subretinal fluid, or subretinal hyperreflective material and/or FFA (leakage classified as subfoveal or as juxtafoveal or extrafoveal)
- Actively treated with aflibercept and given 3 monthly loading doses followed by the treat and extend regime
- Maximal interval period is less than or equal to 8 weekly injections
- Patients must understand and sign the ethics board-approved consent form

Exclusion Criteria
- Ocular criteria:
  - Co-existing retinal and/or macular disease (DME, RVO, high myopia of 8 diopters or more, retinal detachment, macular hole stage 2 or above, significant vitreomacular traction or epiretinal membrane, etc.)
  - Co-existing ocular disease (glaucoma, uveitis, etc.)
  - History of uveitis or intraocular inflammation, scleritis, or episcleritis
  - History of corneal transplant, pars planar vitrectomy, or aphakia
  - History of therapeutic radiation to the region of the study eye
  - Media opacity obstructing investigation or assessment (cataract, corneal scar, vitreous hemorrhage)
  - Treat and extend period beyond 8 weeks
  - Any intravitreal injection of steroid within 3 months before randomization
- Systemic criteria:
  - Poorly controlled systemic disease including hypertension and diabetes
  - Any acute coronary event or stroke within 6 months before randomization
  - Malignancy within 5 years
  - Systemic anti-VEGF treatment
  - Allergy or sensitivity to investigational product, including fluoresceine dye, anesthetics, aflibercept, or brolucizumab

Ages Eligible for Study
50 Years and Older (Adult, Older Adult)

Sexes Eligible for Study
All

Accepts Healthy Volunteers
No

Design Details

Primary Purpose: Treatment
Allocation: Randomized
Interventional Model: Parallel Assignment
Interventional Model Description: Parallel interventional arms with an option of rescue treatment
Masking: Single (Participant)
Masking Description: Patients are randomized and masked from the treatment

Arms and interventions

Participant group/arm	Intervention/treatment
Experimental: Brolucizumab new drug (brolocizumab) and novel treatment protocol	Drug: Brolucizumab • Intravitreal injection • Other Names: –Beovu
Active Comparator: Aflibercept aflibercept and continuing on the traditional T&E protocol. There will also be a rescue option for those in the aflibercept arm who are not responding well to also switch to brolocizumab	Drug: Aflibercept • Intravitreal injection • Other Names: –Eylea

Primary outcome measures

Outcome Measure	Measure description	Time frame
Central Macular thickness	Measurement of the change in macular thickness (μm)	1 year

Secondary outcome measures

Outcome measure	Measure description	Time frame
Visual acuity	Change in best-corrected visual acuity (BCVA), LogMAR	1 year
Treatment interval	Change in the duration of the treatment interval between each injection (weeks)	1 year
Complications	Relating to the drug (e.g., inflammation), relating to the procedure (glaucoma, cataract, retinal detachment, hemorrhage, etc.)	1 year
Optical Coherence Tomography features	Changes and presence of OCT features during every follow-up visit (subretinal fluid, intraretinal fluid, and pigmented epithelial defect)	1 year

Sponsor

The University of Hong Kong

Collaborators

No information provided

Investigators

No information provided

General Publications

- Friedman DS, O'Colmain BJ, Munoz B, Tomany SC, McCarty C, de Jong PT, Nemesure B, Mitchell P, Kempen J; Eye Diseases Prevalence Research Group. Prevalence of age-related macular degeneration in the United States. Arch Ophthalmol. 2004 Apr;122(4):564–72. https://doi.org/10.1001/archopht.122.4.564. Erratum In: Arch Ophthalmol. 2011 Sep;129(9):1188.
- Bressler NM. Age-related macular degeneration is the leading cause of blindness. JAMA. 2004 Apr 21;291(15):1900–1. https://doi.org/10.1001/jama.291.15.1900. No abstract available.
- Wong WL, Su X, Li X, Cheung CM, Klein R, Cheng CY, Wong TY. Global prevalence of age-related macular degeneration and disease burden projection for 2020 and 2040: a systematic review and meta-analysis. Lancet Glob Health. 2014 Feb;2(2):e106–16. https://doi.org/10.1016/S2214-109X(13)70145-1. Epub 2014 Jan 3.
- Cheung CM, Li X, Cheng CY, Zheng Y, Mitchell P, Wang JJ, Wong TY. Prevalence, racial variations, and risk factors of age-related macular degeneration in Singaporean Chinese, Indians, and Malays. Ophthalmology. 2014 Aug;121(8):1598–603. https://doi.org/10.1016/j.ophtha.2014.02.004. Epub 2014 Mar 22.
- Brown DM, Kaiser PK, Michels M, Soubrane G, Heier JS, Kim RY, Sy JP, Schneider S; ANCHOR Study Group. Ranibizumab versus verteporfin for neovascular age-related macular degeneration. N Engl J Med. 2006 Oct 5;355(14):1432–44. https://doi.org/10.1056/NEJMoa062655.
- Rosenfeld PJ, Brown DM, Heier JS, Boyer DS, Kaiser PK, Chung CY, Kim RY; MARINA Study Group. Ranibizumab for neovascular age-related macular degeneration. N Engl J Med. 2006 Oct 5;355(14):1419–31. https://doi.org/10.1056/NEJMoa054481.
- Holz FG, Tadayoni R, Beatty S, Berger A, Cereda MG, Cortez R, Hoyng CB, Hykin P, Staurenghi G, Heldner S, Bogumil T, Heah T, Sivaprasad S. Multicountry real-life experience of anti-vascular endothelial growth factor therapy for wet age-related macular degeneration. Br J Ophthalmol. 2015 Feb;99(2):220–6. https://doi.org/10.1136/bjophthalmol-2014-305327. Epub 2014 Sep 5.
- Wykoff CC, Ou WC, Brown DM, Croft DE, Wang R, Payne JF, Clark WL, Abdelfattah NS, Sadda SR; TREX-AMD Study Group. Randomized Trial of Treat-and-Extend versus Monthly Dosing for Neovascular Age-Related Macular Degeneration: 2-Year Results of the TREX-AMD Study. Ophthalmol Retina. 2017 Jul-Aug;1(4):314–321. https://doi.org/10.1016/j.oret.2016.12.004. Epub 2017 Feb 2.
- Schmidt-Erfurth U, Chong V, Loewenstein A, Larsen M, Souied E, Schlingemann R, Eldem B, Mones J, Richard G, Bandello F; European Society of Retina Specialists. Guidelines for the management of neovascular age-related macular degeneration by the European Society of Retina Specialists (EURETINA). Br J

Ophthalmol. 2014 Sep;98(9):1144–67. https://doi.org/10.1136/bjophthalmol-2014-305702.
- Boulanger-Scemama E, Querques G, About F, Puche N, Srour M, Mane V, Massamba N, Canoui-Poitrine F, Souied EH. Ranibizumab for exudative age-related macular degeneration: A five year study of adherence to follow-up in a real-life setting. J Fr Ophtalmol. 2015 Sep;38(7):620–7. https://doi.org/10.1016/j.jfo.2014.11.015. Epub 2015 Apr 23.
- Dugel PU, Koh A, Ogura Y, Jaffe GJ, Schmidt-Erfurth U, Brown DM, Gomes AV, Warburton J, Weichselberger A, Holz FG; HAWK and HARRIER Study Investigators. HAWK and HARRIER: Phase 3, Multicenter, Randomized, Double-Masked Trials of Brolucizumab for Neovascular Age-Related Macular Degeneration. Ophthalmology. 2020 Jan;127(1):72–84. https://doi.org/10.1016/j.ophtha.2019.04.017. Epub 2019 Apr 12.
- Waizel M, Todorova MG, Masyk M, Wolf K, Rickmann A, Helaiwa K, Blanke BR, Szurman P. Switch to aflibercept or ranibizumab after initial treatment with bevacizumab in eyes with neovascular AMD. BMC Ophthalmol. 2017 May 23;17(1):79. https://doi.org/10.1186/s12886-017-0471-x.
- Bulirsch LM, Sassmannshausen M, Nadal J, Liegl R, Thiele S, Holz FG. Short-term real-world outcomes following intravitreal brolucizumab for neovascular AMD: SHIFT study. Br J Ophthalmol. 2022 Sep;106(9):1288–1294. https://doi.org/10.1136/bjophthalmol-2020-318672. Epub 2021 Apr 12.
- Bilgic A, Kodjikian L, March de Ribot F, Vasavada V, Gonzalez-Cortes JH, Abukashabah A, Sudhalkar A, Mathis T. Real-World Experience with Brolucizumab in Wet Age-Related Macular Degeneration: The REBA Study. J Clin Med. 2021 Jun 23;10(13):2758. https://doi.org/10.3390/jcm10132758.
- Mones J, Srivastava SK, Jaffe GJ, Tadayoni R, Albini TA, Kaiser PK, Holz FG, Korobelnik JF, Kim IK, Pruente C, Murray TG, Heier JS. Risk of Inflammation, Retinal Vasculitis, and Retinal Occlusion-Related Events with Brolucizumab: Post Hoc Review of HAWK and HARRIER. Ophthalmology. 2021 Jul;128(7):1050–1059. https://doi.org/10.1016/j.ophtha.2020.11.011. Epub 2020 Nov 15.
- Baumal CR, Spaide RF, Vajzovic L, Freund KB, Walter SD, John V, Rich R, Chaudhry N, Lakhanpal RR, Oellers PR, Leveque TK, Rutledge BK, Chittum M, Bacci T, Enriquez AB, Sund NJ, Subong ENP, Albini TA. Retinal Vasculitis and Intraocular Inflammation after Intravitreal Injection of Brolucizumab. Ophthalmology. 2020 Oct;127(10):1345–1359. https://doi.org/10.1016/j.ophtha.2020.04.017. Epub 2020 Apr 25.
- Baumal CR, Bodaghi B, Singer M, Tanzer DJ, Seres A, Joshi MR, Feltgen N, Gale R. Expert Opinion on Management of Intraocular Inflammation, Retinal Vasculitis, and Vascular Occlusion after Brolucizumab Treatment. Ophthalmol Retina. 2021 Jun;5(6):519–527. https://doi.org/10.1016/j.oret.2020.09.020. Epub 2020 Sep 29.

China

Recruiting

Study of IBI333 in Subjects with Neovascular Age-Related Macular Degeneration

ClinicalTrials.gov ID NCT05639530

Sponsor Innovent Biologics (Suzhou) Co. Ltd.
Information provided by Innovent Biologics (Suzhou) Co. Ltd. (Responsible Party)
Last Update Posted 2023-03-10

Study Overview

Brief Summary
This study is designed for multi-center, open-label, dose escalation phase I trial to evaluate the safety and tolerability of a single and multiple intravitreal injection of IBI333 in subjects with neovascular age-related macular degeneration (nAMD).

Official Title
A Dose Escalation Phase I Clinical Study to Evaluate the Tolerability and Safety of IBI333 in Subjects with Neovascular Age-related Macular Degeneration (nAMD)

Conditions
Neovascular Age-Related Macular Degeneration

Intervention/Treatment
- Biological: IBI333

Other Study ID Numbers
- CIBI333A101

Study Start (Actual)
2022-11-30

Primary Completion (Estimated)
2023-10-13

Study Completion (Estimated)
2024-01-07

Enrollment (Estimated)
24

Study Type
Interventional

Phase
Phase 1

Study Contact
Name: Youxin Chen, MD
Phone Number: +8613801025972
Email: chenyouxinpumch@163.com
China
Beijing Locations

Beijing, Beijing, China, 101199
Recruiting
Peking Union Medical College Hospital, Chinese Academy of Medical Sciences

Contact
Yanyuan Sun
010-87705665 sunyanyuan@pumch.cn
Principal Investigator:
Hong Dai, MD

Eligibility Criteria
Description

Inclusion Criteria
- Willing and able to sign the informed consent form and comply with visit and study procedures per protocol
- Male or female patients ≥50 yrs. of age
- Active CNV lesions secondary to neovascular AMD
- BCVA score of 19–78 letters using ETDRS charts in the study eye
- Female subjects of childbearing age or male subjects with childbearing age female partners agree to take effective contraceptive measures from the screening period to 6 months after the end of treatment

Exclusion Criteria
- Concomitant diseases that may cause subjects to fail to respond to the treatment or confuse the interpretation of the study results
- Tractional retinal detachment, pre-retinal fibrosis, vitreomacular traction, or epiretinal membrane involving the fovea or disrupting the macular structure in the study eye
- Active ocular or periocular inflammation/infection in either eye
- Prior to any treatment of the following in the study eye:
  - Anti-VEGF therapy within 90 days prior to screening
  - Intraocular glucocorticoid injection within 180 days prior to screening
  - Laser photocoagulation or photodynamic therapy within 90 days prior to screening
  - Intraocular surgery within 90 days prior to screening
  - Laser posterior capsulotomy, laser trabeculectomy, or laser peripheral iridectomy within 30 days prior to screening

- Glycated hemoglobin (HbA1c) > 8% within 28 days prior to screening
- Uncontrolled hypertension (defined as systolic blood pressure > 160 mmHg or diastolic blood pressure > 100 mmHg)
- Systemic administration of steroids within 30 days prior to screening
- Systemic administration of anti-VEGF drugs within 90 days prior to screening
- History of severe hypersensitivity/allergic to active ingredients or any excipients of the study drug, or fluorescein and povidone iodine
- Participated in any clinical study of any other drug within 90 days prior to enrollment or attempted to participate in other drug trials during the study
- Other conditions unsuitable for enrollment as judged by investigators

Ages Eligible for Study
50 Years and Older (Adult, Older Adult)

Sexes Eligible for Study
All

Accepts Healthy Volunteers
No

Design Details
Primary Purpose: Treatment
Allocation: Nonrandomized
Interventional Model: Sequential Assignment
Masking: None (Open Label)

Arms and interventions

Participant group/arm	Intervention/treatment
Experimental: treated with different doses of single intravitreal injections of IBI333 Biological: IBI333 Dose 1 IBI333 of single IVT injections, Biological: IBI333 Dose 2 IBI333 of single IVT injections	Biological: IBI333 • Intravitreal injection of IBI333
Experimental: treated with different doses of multiple intravitreal injections of IBI333 Biological: IBI333 Dose 3 IBI333 of multiple IVT injections, Biological: IBI333 Dose 4 IBI333 of multiple IVT injections	Biological: IBI333 • Intravitreal injection of IBI333

Primary outcome measures

Outcome Measure	Measure description	Time frame
Safety and tolerance indicators	1. Incidence, relatedness, and severity of all adverse events (AE), treatment emergent adverse events (TEAE) and serious adverse events (SAE) 2. Incidence of dose-limiting toxicity	Through study completion, a maximum of 24 weeks

Secondary outcome measures

Outcome measure	Measure description	Time frame
The area under the curve (AUC) of serum concentration of the drug after the administration		Through study completion, a maximum of 24 weeks
Maximum concentration (C_{max}) of the drug after the administration		Through study completion, a maximum of 24 weeks
Time at which maximum concentration (T_{max}) occurs for the drug after the administration		Through study completion, a maximum of 24 weeks
The half-life (t1/2) of drug after the administration		Through study completion, a maximum of 24 weeks
Number of participants with anti-drug antibodies or neutralizing antibodies		Through study completion, a maximum of 24 weeks
Changes of BCVA measured by the ETDRS chart from baseline		Through study completion, a maximum of 24 weeks
Changes of CST measured by spectral domain optical coherence tomography (SD-OCT) from baseline		Through study completion, a maximum of 24 weeks
Proportion of subjects without intraretinal or subretinal fluid on SD-OCT		Through study completion, a maximum of 24 weeks
Change of height of pigment epithelial detachment from baseline on SD-OCT		Through study completion, a maximum of 24 weeks

Sponsor
Innovent Biologics (Suzhou) Co. Ltd.

Collaborators
No information provided

Investigators
No information provided

General Publications
No publications available

China

Recruiting

QA108 Phase II Study in Subjects with Intermediate Age-Related Macular Degeneration

ClinicalTrials.gov ID NCT05562219

Sponsor Smilebiotek Zhuhai Limited
Information provided by Smilebiotek Zhuhai Limited (Responsible Party)
Last Update Posted 2022-09-30

Study Overview

Brief Summary
This is a phase 2, randomized, double-masked, placebo-controlled, multicenter study. To evaluate the efficacy and safety of QA108 granules in the treatment of intermediate age-related macular degeneration.

Detailed Description
Approximately 12 sites will randomize a total of approximately 120 subjects. The subject randomization code table is generated using block randomization. Randomization of not less than 120 cases receiving treatment (treatment and placebo groups) at a ratio of 1:1 for the treatment and control groups.

Clinic study visits will occur on Day -7 to Day -1 (Screening/Baseline) (Randomization); Treatment Visits for weeks 4, 8, 12,16,20, and 24 (all ±3 days); sites will contact each subject to update the efficacy date and adverse events (AEs) and review concomitant medications (CMs).

Official Title
A Randomized, Double-Masked, Placebo-Controlled, Multicenter, Phase II Clinical Study of the Efficacy and Safety of QA108 Granules in the Treatment of Intermediate Age-Related Macular Degeneration

Conditions
Intermediate Age-Related Macular Degeneration

Intervention/Treatment
- Drug: QA108 granules
- Drug: QA108 granules placebo

Other Study ID Numbers
- QA108

Study Start (Actual)
2022-06-29

Primary Completion (Estimated)
2024-03-30

Study Completion (Estimated)
2024-07-31

Enrollment (Estimated)
120

Study Type
Interventional

Phase
Phase 2

Study Contact
Name: youxin chen
Phone Number: 010-6915 6351
Email: chenyouxinpumch@163.com
China

Peking, China
Recruiting
Peking Union Medical College Hospital (PUMCH)

Contact
youxin chen
010 6915 6351 chenyouxinpumch@163.com

Eligibility Criteria
Description

Inclusion Criteria
- The study eye is diagnosed by Western medicine with intermediate age-related macular degeneration, i.e., at least one large drusen (≥ 125 μm in diameter) is visible within two papillary diameters (PD) away from the fovea
- Consistent with the TCM diagnosis of the type of Yang-hyperactivity due to Yin-deficiency
- Age 45–85 years old (both inclusive), male or female
- The study eye has a BCVA of 83-34 ETDRS letters (inclusive), which is equivalent to a Snellen visual acuity of 20/25 to 20/200 (inclusive)
- The subject is voluntary to participate in this clinical study, provide informed consent, and sign the informed consent form

Exclusion Criteria
- The study eye is with concomitant eye disorders that may interfere with the observation of the trial as judged by the investigator, including pathological myopia, glaucoma, diabetic retinopathy, retinal vein occlusion, uveitis, retinal detachment, optic neuropathy (optic neuritis, atrophy, papilledema), and macular hole
- The study eye has an intraocular pressure (IOP) ≥ 25 mmHg
- The study eye is presented with GA

- Previous ophthalmic surgery in the study eye: vitrectomy and macular translocation
- Aphakia (except pseudophakia) or posterior capsule rupture (except YAG laser posterior capsulotomy after IOL implantation at more than 1 month prior to screening) of the study eye
- Any intraocular or periocular surgery of the study eye and intraocular surgery (except eyelid surgery) of the nonstudy eye within 3 months
- The study eye is diagnosed with cataract affecting fundus observation, which may require cataract surgery within 6 months at the discretion of the investigator
- The study eye has received the following treatment within 3 months prior to screening: macular laser photocoagulation and micro-pulse laser therapy
- The patient received relevant TCM treatment within 1 month prior to screening
- Active ocular infection in either eye
- The nonstudy eye has a BCVA of less than 19 ETDRS letters (not inclusive)
- Known allergy to the therapeutic or diagnostic drug used in the study protocol, including the single drug components in the study drugs
- Poorly controlled hypertension (systolic blood pressure $\geq$ 160 mmHg or diastolic blood pressure $\geq$ 100 mmHg after regular use of antihypertensive drugs)
- Patients with platelet count $\leq 100 \times 10^9$/L, total bilirubin (TBIL) > upper limit of normal (ULN), alanine transaminase (ALT), or aspartate aminotransferase (AST) > 1.5 × ULN, and blood creatinine > ULN
- Pregnant women, women who are breastfeeding, those who plan for pregnancy in the next six months, or those who are unwilling to take effective birth controls during the study course and until six months after drug withdrawal
- Any uncontrollable clinical disorder prior to the start of treatment, such as severe psychiatric, neurological, respiratory, immunological, hematological, and cardiac system diseases, and malignant tumors
- Subjects who have participated in other clinical trials within 3 months prior to this trial
- Patients who are unsuitable for participating at the discretion of the investigator

Ages Eligible for Study
45 Years to 85 Years (Adult, Older Adult)

Sexes Eligible for Study
All

Accepts Healthy Volunteers
No

Design Details
Primary Purpose: Treatment
Allocation: Randomized
Interventional Model: Parallel Assignment
Masking: Quadruple (Participant Care Provider Investigator Outcomes Assessor)

Arms and interventions

Participant group/arm	Intervention/treatment
Experimental: Treatment group (QA108 granules) QA108 granules, 7.5 g/bag, 2 bags/time, BID	Drug: QA108 granules • Take the medication as required for 24 weeks
Placebo Comparator: Placebo group (QA108 granule simulants) QA108 granule simulants, 7.5 g/bag, 2 bags/time, BID	Drug: QA108 granules placebo • Take the medication as required for 24 weeks

Primary outcome measures

Outcome measure	Measure description	Time frame
Percentage change from baseline in the drusen area	1. Change from baseline in the drusen area as measured by optical coherence tomography (OCT) 2. Assessments will be conducted by the central reading center (CRC)	Weeks 24

Secondary outcome measures

Outcome measure	Measure description	Time frame
Percentage change from baseline in the drusen area	Change from baseline in the drusen area as measured by optical coherence tomography (OCT)	Weeks 4,8,12,16, and 20

Sponsor
Smilebiotek Zhuhai Limited

Collaborators
No information provided

Investigators
No information provided

General Publications
No publications available

Italy

Recruiting

Photobiomodulation in Dry Age-Related Macular Degeneration (DRUSEN)

ClinicalTrials.gov ID NCT06046118

Sponsor Azienda Ospedaliera Universitaria Mater Domini, Catanzaro
Information provided by Giuseppe Giannaccare, Azienda Ospedaliera Universitaria Mater Domini, Catanzaro (Responsible Party)
Last Update Posted 2023-09-21

Study Overview

Brief Summary

The goal of this clinical trial is to evaluate the effects of consecutive Yellow and Red Light Emitting Diode photobiomodulation in dry age-related macular degeneration (AMD). The main questions it aims to answer are:

- Is Yellow and Red Light Emitting Diode photobiomodulation effective in decreasing drusen volume in patients affected by dry AMD?
- Does Yellow and Red Light Emitting Diode photobiomodulation increase visual acuity and contrast sensitivity in patients affected by dry AMD? Participants will be randomly assigned to a treatment or a sham group

Treatment consists of two cycles with two phases each:

- first phase: 300 seconds of continuous Yellow light with eyes closed +60 seconds of pulsed Yellow light with eyes opened
- 2d phase: 300 seconds of continuous Red light with eyes closed +60 seconds of pulsed Red light with eyes opened

Cycle 1 consists of 8 sessions (two PBM per week for 4 weeks) and cycle 2 consists of 6 sessions (two PBM per week for 3 weeks).

Researchers will compare patients in the treatment group to those in the sham group to evaluate differences in objective signs and subjective symptoms of dry AMD.

Official Title

Outcomes of Photobiomodulation in DRy AgeRelated macUlar Degeneration: a proSpective multicEnter raNdomized Controlled (DRUSEN) Study

Conditions

Age-Related Macular Degeneration

Intervention/Treatment

- Device: Yellow and red light emitting diode photobiomodulation (Eye Light, Espansione Group, Bologna, Italy)
- Device: Sham Mask

Other Study ID Numbers

- PBM AMD

Study Start (Actual)

2023-04-01

Primary Completion (Estimated)

2024-12-31

Study Completion (Estimated)

2024-12-31

Enrollment (Estimated)
180

Study Type
Interventional

Phase
Not Applicable

Study Contact
Name: Giuseppe Giannaccare
Phone Number: 003909613647135
Email: giuseppe.giannaccare@unicz.it
France

Paris, France
Recruiting
University of Paris

Contact
Pierre Raphael Rothschild

Contact
Federico Bernabei
federico.bernabei89@gmail.com

Italy

Ferrara, Italy
Recruiting
Università degli Studi di Ferrara

Contact
Massimo Busin

Contact
Marco Pellegrini
marco.pellegrini@hotmail.it

Napoli, Italy
Recruiting
Università degli studi della Campania Luigi Vanvitelli

Contact
Claudio Iovino
claudioiovino88@gmail.com

Contact
Francesca Simonelli

Torino, Italy
Recruiting
Università di Torino

Contact
Michele Reibaldi

Contact
Enrico Borrelli
borrelli.enrico@yahoo.com

Turkey

Ankara, Turkey
Recruiting
University of Ankara

Contact
Sibel Demirel
drsibeldemireltr@yahoo.com.tr

Koç, Turkey
Recruiting
Koç University Hospital

Contact
Murat Murat Hasanreisoğlu
drhasanreisoglu@gmail.com

United Kingdom

Taunton, United Kingdom
Recruiting
Earlam and Christopher

Contact
Sarah Farrant
sarahfarrant@gmail.com

Eligibility Criteria
Description

Inclusion Criteria
- BCVA ETDRS >40 L ETDRS at 4 meters
- Diagnosis of DRY AMD AREDS grades 2–3
- Ability to communicate well with the investigator and able to understand and comply with the requirements of the study

Exclusion Criteria
- Concomitant epilepsy
- Neurological diseases
- Psychiatric pathologies
- Herpes virus infections
- Dense cataract

- Pregnancy
- Other significant ocular and/or retinal diseases

Ages Eligible for Study
50 Years and Older (Adult, Older Adult)

Sexes Eligible for Study
All

Accepts Healthy Volunteers
No

Design Details
Primary Purpose: Treatment
Allocation: Randomized
Interventional Model: Parallel Assignment
Masking: Double (Participant Investigator)

Arms and interventions

Participant group/arm	Intervention/treatment
Experimental: Treatment group Two cycles of treatment using continuous and pulsed yellow light followed by continuous and pulsed red light Cycle 1 consists of 8 sessions (two sessions per week for 4 weeks) and cycle 2 consists of 6 sessions (two sessions per week for 3 weeks)	Device: Yellow and red light emitting diode photobiomodulation (Eye Light, Espansione Group, Bologna, Italy) • Each session consists of: – first phase: 300 seconds of continuous Yellow light (eyes closed) + 60 seconds of pulsed Yellow light (eyes opened) – second phase: 300 seconds of continuous Red light(eyes closed) + 60 seconds of pulsed Red light (eyes opened) Cycle 1: 8 sessions (two PBM per week for 4 weeks) Cycle 2: 6 sessions (two PBM per week for 3 weeks)
Sham Comparator: Sham group Sham treatment will occur using a sham mask, designed to release a very low level of light, in this way the patient will not be able to distinguish if he is receiving the treatment or not Cycle 1 consists of 8 sessions (two sessions per week for 4 weeks) and cycle 2 consists of 6 sessions (two sessions per week for 3 weeks)	Device: Sham Mask • Low light emission mask (Sham Mask, Espansione group, Bologna, Italy)

Primary outcome measures

Outcome measure	Measure description	Time frame
Best Corrected Visual Acuity variation	ETDRS letters	1 month, 2 months, and 4 months after each cycle
Drusen Volume Variation	Based on SD-OCT Heidelberg	1 month, 2 months, and 4 months after each cycle
Contrast sensitivity variation	Based on Pelli Robson chart	1 month, 2 months, and 4 months after each cycle

Sponsor
Azienda Ospedaliera Universitaria Mater Domini, Catanzaro

Collaborators
No information provided

Investigators
No information provided

General Publications
No publications available

Korea

Recruiting

Study of Application of Transcutaneous Pulsed Electrical Stimulation Around Eye in Age-Related Macular Degeneration

ClinicalTrials.gov ID NCT05259371

Sponsor Nu Eyne Co., Ltd.
Information provided by Nu Eyne Co., Ltd. (Responsible Party)
Last Update Posted 2023-09-11

Study Overview

Brief Summary
This study aims to evaluate the safety and efficacy of applying pulse electrical stimulation around the eyes of age-related macular patients.

Detailed Description
Duration of study period (per participant): Screening period (0–4 weeks), Intervention period (16 weeks). Patient needs to visit site at least 5 times (Screening, V2, V3, V4, V5). V2 can be done with screening visit. Visits 3, 4, 5 is 2 weeks, 6 weeks, and 16 weeks after visit 2 (Baseline).

Official Title
A 16-Week, Multi-Center, Open-Label, Exploratory Study to Evaluate the Safety and Efficacy of the Application of Pulse Electrical Stimulation Around the Eye in Early to Moderate Dry Age-Related Macular Degeneration

Conditions
Early to Moderate Dry Age-Related Macular Degeneration

Intervention/Treatment
- Drug: Transcutaneous Pulsed Electrical Stimulation (Device: Nu Eyne M02)

Other Study ID Numbers
- NE_RTN_002

Study Start (Actual)
2022-10-05

Primary Completion (Estimated)
2024-06-30

Study Completion (Estimated)
2024-06-30

Enrollment (Estimated)
25

Study Type
Interventional

Phase
Not Applicable

Study Contact
Name: Jinho Jung, Ph.D. candidate
Phone Number: +821083113509
Email: jinho.jung@nueyne.com

Study Contact Backup
Name: Nayoung Kang
Phone Number: +821073734097
Email: nayoung.kang@nueyne.com
Korea, Republic of

Seoul, Korea, Republic of, 05505
Recruiting
Asan Medical Center

Contact
Yoon Jeon Kim, M.D., Ph.D.

Principal Investigator:
Yoon Jeon Kim, M.D., Ph.D.

Seoul, Korea, Republic of, 06192
Not yet recruiting
Nune Eye Hospital

Contact
Jong Min Kim, M.D., MS.

Principal Investigator:
Jong Min Kim, M.D., MS.

Gyeonggi-do Locations

Ansan, Gyeonggi-do, Korea, Republic of, 15355
Recruiting
Korea University Ansan Hospital

Contact
Cheol Min Yun, M.D., Ph.D.

Principal Investigator:
Cheol Min Yun, M.D., Ph.D.

Eligibility Criteria
Description

Inclusion Criteria

- 50 years or older
- Has a confirmed diagnosis of early to moderate AMD
  - According to Staging of age-related macular degeneration of the Beckman Initiative for the Macular Research Classification Committee

    early AMD: Medium drusen (>63 μm; ≤125 μm) and No AMD pigmentary abnormalities
    moderate AMD: Large drusen (>125 μm) and/or Any AMD pigmentary abnormalities

- Best Corrected Visual Acuity [BCVA] of 20/200 or better measured by Early Treatment Diabetic Retinopathy Study (ETDRS) Charts
- A person who voluntarily agreed to participate in this clinical trial

Exclusion Criteria

- Subject who is observed to have atrophy of 175 micrometers or more in diameter invading the fovea on fundus examination or fundus autofluorescent with more than one eye
- Subject who is observed to have exudative macular degeneration on fundus examination or optical coherence tomography (OCT) with more than one eye
- Has a history of intravitreal injection, laser treatment, etc.
- Has eye pathology other than early age-related macular degeneration that may affect the outcome of clinical trials
- Has a history of vitrectomy due to macular disease or cataract surgery within 1 month
- Has a disease that is judged to be difficult to interpret in an ophthalmic imaging examination due to ocular media opacity
- Has a history of uncontrollable systemic chronic disease (diabetes mellitus) or malignancy (cases that have not recurred for more than 5 years after complete recovery are excluded)
- Autoimmune disease (Sjögren's syndrome, Rheumatoid arthritis, systemic lupus erythematosus, Graves' disease, etc.)

- Has a severe hearing impairment
- A person who is sensitive to orbit nerve stimulation and cannot be treated
- Has a history of substance and/or alcohol abuse
- Has a confirmed diagnosis of psychiatric disease (depression, schizophrenia, bipolar disorder, dementia, etc.)
- Those who participated in other clinical trials within 30 days of the screening visit
- Those who are judged to have "other reasons for prohibition of use" of our clinical trial medical device: heart-related problems and seizure. Patients transplanted metal or electronic devices in the head and neck including deep brain stimulation devices. Patients suffering from unknown pain. Patients with implantable or wearable cardioverter defibrillator. Patients who are warned not to use clinical trial devices or are prohibited from using them (dental implants are accepted)
- In the case of subjects judged by the researcher that it would be difficult to participate in clinical trials
- Among female subjects who are likely to be pregnant, those who disagree to contraception in a medically permitted manner during this clinical trial period
  - Medically permitted contraception: condom, Oral contraception that lasted for at least 3 months, contraceptive injection, contraceptive implant, intrauterine device, etc.

Ages Eligible for Study
50 Years and Older (Adult, Older Adult)

Sexes Eligible for Study
All

Accepts Healthy Volunteers
No

Design Details
Primary Purpose: Treatment
Allocation: N/A
Interventional Model: Single Group Assignment
Interventional Model Description: • Experimental: Transcutaneous Pulsed Electrical Stimulation Treatment Patients wear our clinical trial device 30 mins once a day for 16 weeks. Device: Nu eyne M02
Masking: None (Open Label)

Arms and interventions

Participant group/arm	Intervention/treatment
Experimental: Transcutaneous Pulsed Electrical Stimulation Treatment Patients wear our clinical trial device 30 mins once a day for 16 weeks. Device: Nu eyne M02	Drug: Transcutaneous Pulsed Electrical Stimulation (Device: Nu Eyne M02) • Pulse Electrical Stimulation Patients wear our clinical trial device 30 mins once a day for 16 weeks

Primary outcome measures

Outcome measure	Measure description	Time frame
Number of Safety Events	Check the safety issues (AE, SAE, etc.)	baseline ~16 weeks

Secondary outcome measures

Outcome measure	Measure description	Time frame
Changes in contrast sensitivity	Check the change of contrast sensitivity in the baseline, 6, and 16 weeks	baseline, 6, 16 weeks
Changes in score of VFQ-25(National Eye Institute)	Check the change of Changes in score of VFQ-25 (National Eye Institute) in the baseline, 6, 1and 6 weeks	baseline, 6, 16 weeks
Changes in best corrected visual acuity (Early Treatment Diabetic Retinopathy Study (ETDRS) Chart)	Check the change of best-corrected visual acuity in the baseline, 6, and 16 weeks	baseline, 6, 16 weeks
Changes in drusen area using optical coherence tomography (OCT)	Check the change of drusen area using optical coherence tomography (OCT) in the baseline, 6, and 16 weeks	baseline, 6, 16 weeks
Changes in drusen volume using optical coherence tomography (OCT)	Check the change of drusen volume using optical coherence tomography (OCT) in the baseline, 6, and 16 weeks	baseline, 6, 16 weeks
Progression to advanced Age-related Macular Degeneration (AMD) using fundus autofluorescence (FAF)	Check the Progression to advanced Age-related Macular Degeneration (AMD) using fundus autofluorescence (FAF) in the baseline, 6, and 16 weeks	baseline, 6, 16 weeks
Progression to advanced Age-related Macular Degeneration (AMD) using fundus photography	Check the Progression to advanced Age-related Macular Degeneration (AMD) using fundus photography in the baseline, 6, and 16 weeks	baseline, 6, 16 weeks

Sponsor
Nu Eyne Co., Ltd.

Collaborators
No information provided

Investigators
No information provided

General Publications
No publications available

Norway

Not Yet Recruiting

Photobiomodulation for Dry Age-Related Macular Degeneration

ClinicalTrials.gov ID NCT05507840

Sponsor Oslo University Hospital
Information provided by ANCA ROALD, Oslo University Hospital (Responsible Party)
Last Update Posted 2022-10-12

Study Overview

Brief Summary
The study will investigate the effect of photobiomodulation treatment on the risk of developing late age-related macular degeneration (AMD) in the study eye in patients with wet AMD in the fellow eye.

Official Title
Photobiomodulation for Dry Age-Related Macular Degeneration

Conditions
Photobiomodulation
Age-Related Macular Degeneration

Intervention/Treatment
- Device: Valeda machine

Other Study ID Numbers
- 456056
- Study Start (Estimated)
- 2022-12-01

Primary Completion (Estimated)
2026-12-01

Study Completion (Estimated)
2027-12-01

Enrollment (Estimated)
121

Study Type
Interventional

Phase
Not Applicable
No location data

Eligibility Criteria
Description

Inclusion Criteria
- Patients with dry AMD in the study eye and wet AMD in the control eye

Exclusion Criteria
- Geographic atrophy of the central macular region at enrolment
- Previous/active wet AMD in the study eye
- A history of epilepsy
- Retinal diseases apart from AMD
- Significant media opacities
- Cataracts worse than grade 2 (LOCS III classification)
- Change in AREDS 2 supplements (vitamins) 1 month before the study and during the study trial was allowed
- Ongoing systemic medications that are photosensitizing (e.g., tetracyclins)
- Systemic medications during the last 6 months that can cause deposits in the macular region (hydroxychloroquine, amiodarone)
- Unable to give informed consent
- Unable to cooperate with the treatment and follow-up

Ages Eligible for Study
50 Years and Older (Adult, Older Adult)

Sexes Eligible for Study
All

Accepts Healthy Volunteers
No
Study Plan

Design Details
Primary Purpose: Treatment
Allocation: Randomized
Interventional Model: Parallel Assignment
Masking: Double (Participant Care Provider)

Arms and interventions

Participant group/arm	Intervention/treatment
Experimental: Intervention Near or infrared light provided by the Valeda machine will be applied in the intervention eye	Device: Valeda machine • Photobiomodulation treatment with Valeda machine will be applied every six months for 2 years in patients with dry age-related macular degeneration
Sham Comparator: Control Light with very low intensity provided by the same Valeda machine will be applied in the control eye	Device: Valeda machine • Photobiomodulation treatment with the Valeda machine will be applied every six months for 2 years in patients with dry age-related macular degeneration

Primary outcome measures

Outcome measure	Measure description	Time frame
Percentage of patients who develop late AMD in the study eye compared with control after 3 years of follow-up		3 years

Sponsor
Oslo University Hospital

Collaborators
No information provided

Investigators
No information provided

General Publications
No publications available

South America

Recruiting

OcuDyne System in the Treatment of AMD

ClinicalTrials.gov ID NCT05091476

Sponsor OcuDyne, Inc.
Information provided by OcuDyne, Inc. (Responsible Party)
Last Update Posted 2023-08-24

Study Overview

Brief Summary
Feasibility of the OcuDyne OPTiC System in patients with late-stage nonexudative age-related macular degeneration.

Detailed Description
This study evaluates the safety and feasibility of using the OcuDyne OPTiC System in patients with late-stage nonexudative age-related macular degeneration.

Official Title
A Clinical Study to Evaluate the Safety and Feasibility of the OcuDyne System in the Treatment of Age-Related Macular Degeneration (AMD)

Conditions
Age-Related Macular Degeneration

Intervention/Treatment
- Device: OPTiC System

Other Study ID Numbers
- OC-1901AR

Study Start (Actual)
2022-07-25

Primary Completion (Estimated)
2024-04-30

Study Completion (Estimated)
2024-04-30

Enrollment (Estimated)
20

Study Type
Interventional

Phase
Not Applicable

Study Contact
Name: Luana R Wilbur, BS
Phone Number: 858-442-7178
Email: lwilbur@ocudyne.com
Argentina

Buenos Aires, Argentina
Recruiting
Buenos Aires Macula

Contact
Agustina Goyret
+541123192313 agoyret@bamsite.com.ar

Buenos Aires, Argentina
Recruiting
ENERI

Contact
Matias Correa
541149747373 mcorrea@bioscienceweb.com

Eligibility Criteria
Description

Inclusion Criteria
- Must be able to understand and provide informed consent on an Independent Ethics Committee (EC) approved informed consent form (ICF)
- Must be willing and able to return for scheduled treatment and follow-up examinations for up to a 7-month duration

- Adults at least 60 years of age at the time of consent
- Diagnosed with nonexudative Age-Related Macular Degeneration with current or previous evidence of at least one large drusen (measuring 125 microns or greater) and nascent geographic atrophy (nGA) or GA in the study eye
- ETDRS best-corrected visual acuity (BCVA) letter score of less than 56 letters (Snellen equivalent of 20/80 or worse) in the study eye, which in the Investigator's judgment is caused by nonexudative age-related macular degeneration (AMD)
- The confirmed presence of ophthalmic artery (OA) stenosis (leading to the study eye)

Exclusion Criteria
Ocular

- Any surgical intraocular treatment (including laser) within 3 months in the study eye
- History of exudative AMD or Anti-Vascular Endothelial Growth Factor (anti-VEGF) injections within 6 months in the study eye
- Presence of ocular media affecting visual acuity or the ability to visualize the retina in either eye (e.g., central corneal scarring, lens opacities along the visual axis, posterior capsule opacification, etc.)
- History of chronic, recurring inflammatory eye disease in either eye (e.g., scleritis, uveitis, corneal edema, etc.)
- Presence of diabetic retinopathy in either eye
- Evidence of macular edema secondary to exudation in the study eye
- History of amaurosis fugax, central or retinal artery or vein occlusion, anterior ischemic optic neuropathy (AION) or nonarteritic anterior ischemic optic neuropathy (NAION) or any diagnosis of a macular disease other than AMD such as Stargardt disease, cone rod dystrophy, angioid streaks, or toxic maculopathies such as Plaquenil maculopathy
- Myopia >6.0 Diopters (D) spherical equivalent (SE) or Axial Length ≥ 26.0 mm in the study eye
- Presence of visually significant epiretinal membrane in the study eye
- Participation in any eye-related drug or device clinical trial involving either eye within 90 days prior to enrolling in this study and/or during study participation

Nonocular

- Any condition that prohibits the use of intravenous contrast agents (e.g., renal insufficiency, previous anaphylactoid reaction to contrast material, treatment with nephrotoxic agents, etc.)
- Previous stroke, including ischemic, hemorrhagic, or transient ischemic attack (TIA)
- Previous myocardial infarction (MI), including ST segment elevation (STEMI), non-ST segment elevation (NSTEMI), or coronary spasm/angina
- Coronary or other intravascular percutaneous procedure, including balloon angioplasty, stent, or filter placement within the last 6 months

- Complete occlusion of the ophthalmic artery
- Pacemaker, Cochlear, or neurostimulation implant
- Presence of cranial aneurysm, clinically significant stenosis in the common carotid artery or internal carotid artery, or tortuous vascular anatomy as seen on pre-procedural CT Angiogram that, in the clinical judgement of the investigator, represents an unreasonable risk to perform the intervention
- Condition associated with increased bleeding risk including but not limited to: major surgical procedure or trauma within 30 days of screening; clinically significant gastrointestinal bleeding within 1 year of screening; known gastric or duodenal ulcer; history of intracranial or spinal bleeding; chronic hemorrhagic disorder; treatment with oral anticoagulant medications (e.g., Warfarin/non-vitamin K anticoagulants [NOACs] exclusionary; aspirin or clopidogrel allowed), known intracranial neoplasm, arteriovenous malformation, or aneurysm
- Treatment with oral anticoagulant medications (e.g., Warfarin/non-vitamin K anticoagulants [NOACs] exclusionary; aspirin or clopidogrel allowed)
- Sustained and uncontrolled hypertension with systolic blood pressure > 180 mmHg
- Diagnosis of moderate to severe symptomatic congestive heart failure (CHF) or chronic obstructive pulmonary disease (COPD)
- Diagnosis of connective tissue, demyelinating, autoimmune, or inflammatory diseases (e.g., lupus, rheumatoid arthritis, scleroderma, giant cell arteritis, multiple sclerosis, etc.)
- Intolerance of either pre- or post- procedure medication regimen
- Pregnancy, lactation, or plans to become pregnant during participation in this clinical trial
- Participation in any other noneye related drug or device clinical trial within 30 days prior to enrolling in this study and/or during study participation

Other

- Use of facial fillers or paralytic drugs during study participation
- Subject who, in the clinical judgement of the investigator, is not otherwise suitable for participation in the study for another clinical reason, as documented by the investigator

Ages Eligible for Study
60 Years and Older (Adult, Older Adult)

Sexes Eligible for Study
All

Accepts Healthy Volunteers
No

Design Details
Primary Purpose: Treatment
Allocation: Nonrandomized
Interventional Model: Single Group Assignment
Masking: None (Open Label)

Arms and interventions

Participant group/arm	Intervention/treatment
Experimental: Eyes treated with the OPTiC System Eyes that OPTiC System treatment has been completed	Device: OPTiC System • OPTiC System procedure
No Intervention: Fellow Eye Contralateral comparator	

Primary outcome measures

Outcome measure	Measure description	Time frame
Adverse Events	Procedural Complications and Adverse Events	Intraoperative through Week 4 postoperative

Sponsor
OcuDyne, Inc.

Collaborators
No information provided

Investigators
- Study Director: Luana R Wilbur, BS, OcuDyne VP, Clinical and Regulatory Affairs

General Publications
No publications available

Thailand

Recruiting

A Study to Investigate the Effect on Central Macular Thickness of Treatment with MG-O-1002 Eye Drops in Participants Aged over 45 with Neovascular Age-Related Macular Degeneration (nAMD)

ClinicalTrials.gov ID NCT05390840

Sponsor Theratocular Biotek Co.
Information provided by Metagone Biotech Inc. (Theratocular Biotek Co.) (Responsible Party)
Last Update Posted 2023-10-19

Study Overview

Brief Summary
A 2 parts Phase II study to investigate the effect on central macular thickness of treatment with MG-O-1002 eye drops in participants aged over 45 with neovascular age-related macular degeneration (nAMD)

Detailed Description
Neovascular Age-related Macular Degeneration (nAMD) is a serious eye disease and a leading cause of irreversible blindness primarily in the older population. Current treatment with anti-vascular endothelial growth factor (VEGF), while effective, requires intravitreal injection meaning administration that needs to be performed by a specialist ophthalmologist and carries procedural risks. MG-O-1002 can be administered as a topical eye drop providing a potentially safer option that can be self-administered increasing accessibility. This study will evaluate the efficacy and safety of topical ocular use of MG-O-1002 in participants with nAMD.

Official Title
A Phase II Trial to Evaluate the Efficacy and Safety of Topical Ocular MG-O-1002 in Patients with Neovascular Age-Related Macular Degeneration (nAMD)

Conditions
Age-Related Macular Degeneration

Intervention/Treatment
- Drug: MG-O-1002
- Other: Placebo

Other Study ID Numbers
- TO-02C201

Study Start (Actual)
2022-08-09

Primary Completion (Estimated)
2023-12

Study Completion (Estimated)
2023-12

Enrollment (Estimated)
36

Study Type
Interventional

Phase
Phase 2

Study Contact
Name: William Chen
Phone Number: 2-2790-6566 ext +886
Email: william.chen@metagone.com.tw

Study Contact Backup
Name: Samjay Lin
Phone Number: 2-2790-6566 ext +886
Email: samjay@metagone.com.tw
Thailand

Bangkok, Thailand
Recruiting
Rajavithi Hospital

Bangkok, Thailand
Recruiting
Ramathibodi Hospital

Khon Kaen, Thailand
Recruiting
Srinagarind Hospital

Nakhon Pathom, Thailand
Recruiting
Metta Pracharak Hospital

Pathum Thani, Thailand
Recruiting
Thammasat University Hospital

Phitsanulok, Thailand
Recruiting
Naresuan University Hospital

Eligibility Criteria
Description

Inclusion Criteria
Part 1:

- Adults aged 45 years or older with a diagnosis of nAMD
- Diagnosis in the study eye of active, pathologic, newly diagnosed, and treatment naïve (i.e., no previous anti-VEGF treatment or other surgery in the study eye)
- Visual acuity from 20/25 to 20/200 in the study eye
- Total lesion size (including neovascularization, blood) $\leqq$ 12 disc areas (30.5 mm2) as assessed by fluorescein angiography
- Demonstrate the ability, or have a family member who is willing and able to, instill topical ocular drops in the study eye
- Ability to give written informed consent and comply with study procedures

Part 2:

- Adults aged 45 years or older with a diagnosis of nAMD
- Participant with nAMD previously treated with 3 injections of Aflibercept within the preceding 4 months, and received the last injection within 30 to 21 days before visit 1 of this study
- Demonstrate the ability, or have a family member who is willing and able to, instill topical ocular drops in the study eye
- Ability to give written informed consent and comply with study procedures

Exclusion Criteria

Part 1:

- Prior use within the last 2 months, or a high possibility of requiring treatment with anti-VEGF therapy (except the study drug) in both eyes during the study
- Abnormal regions identified by Fundus Autofluorescence (FAF) and Optical Coherence Tomography (OCT) involving the center of the fovea are caused by retinal pigment epithelium (RPE) atrophy, RPE tear, photoreceptor attenuation, or fibrosis/scar tissue
- Significant retinal serous pigment epithelial detachment (PED) involving the fovea
- History of, or current clinical evidence in the study eye of aphakia, diabetic macular edema, any ocular inflammation or infection, pathological myopia, retinal detachment, advanced glaucoma, and/or significant media opacity, including cataract
- History or evidence of the following surgeries in the study eye: penetrating keratoplasty or vitrectomy; corneal transplant; corneal or intraocular surgery within 3 months of Screening
- Uncontrolled hypertension despite the use of antihypertensive medications
- Diagnosis of Type 1 or Type 2 diabetes
- Use of medications that in the opinion of the Investigator could interfere with study results
- Participation in any investigational drug or device study, systemic or ocular, within the past 3 months
- Women who are pregnant or breastfeeding
- Women of child-bearing potential who are not using an effective form of birth control
- Known serious allergies or hypersensitivity to the fluorescein dye used in angiography, or to the components of the MG-O-1002 formulation, or to topical anesthetics
- In the opinion of the investigator, a subject who is not suitable for or not likely to be benefited from the study treatment

Part 2:

- More than 30 days between third injection of Aflibercept and Visit 1
- Patients who have received 3 injections of Aflibercept within the last 3 months and need continued treatment in the fellow eye
- Significant retinal serous pigment epithelial detachment (PED), atrophy, or fibrosis/scar involving the fovea
- History or evidence of the following surgeries in the study eye: penetrating keratoplasty or vitrectomy; corneal transplant; corneal or intraocular surgery within 3 months of Screening
- Active intraocular inflammation or uveitis or scleritis or episcleritis in the study eye or ocular or periocular infection in either eye
- Uncontrolled hypertension despite the use of antihypertensive medications

- Diagnosis of Type 1 or Type 2 diabetes
- Use of medications that in the opinion of the Investigator could interfere with study results
- Participation in any investigational drug or device study, systemic or ocular, within the past 3 months
- Women who are pregnant or breastfeeding
- Women of child-bearing potential who are not using an effective form of birth control
- Known serious allergies or hypersensitivity to the fluorescein dye used in angiography, or to the components of the MG-O-1002 formulation, or to topical anesthetics
- In the opinion of the investigator, a subject who is not suitable for or not likely to be benefited from the study treatment

Ages Eligible for Study
45 Years and Older (Adult, Older Adult)

Sexes Eligible for Study
All

Accepts Healthy Volunteers
No

Design Details
Primary Purpose: Treatment
Allocation: Randomized
Interventional Model: Parallel Assignment
Masking: Single (Participant)
Masking Description: Part 1—Open Label (24 Participants); Part 2—Single-Blind to Participant (12 Participants)

Arms and interventions

Participant group/arm	Intervention/treatment
Experimental: Part 1 (MG-O-1002) Drug: MG-O-1002; Dose level: 0.8%; Dosage form: ophthalmic solution; Route of administration: topical ocular	Drug: MG-O-1002 • MG-O-1002 ophthalmic solution in one concentration (0.8%) ocular administration 3 drops in the study eye
Placebo Comparator: Part 2 (MG-O-1002 or Placebo) Arm 1: Drug: MG-O-1002; Dose level: 0.8%; Dosage form: ophthalmic solution; Route of administration: topical ocular Arm 2: Drug: Placebo; Dosage form: ophthalmic solution; Route of administration: topical ocular	Drug: MG-O-1002 • MG-O-1002 ophthalmic solution in one concentration (0.8%) ocular administration 3 drops in the study eye Other: Placebo • The placebo is 0.9% saline ocular administration 3 drops in the study eye

Primary outcome measures

Outcome Measure	Measure description	Time frame
Mean change from baseline in central macular thickness over 12 weeks		up to 12 weeks

Secondary outcome measures

Outcome measure	Measure description	Time frame
Mean change from baseline in Best-Corrected Visual Acuity over 12 weeks		up to 12 weeks
Mean Change from baseline in Visual Field over 12 weeks		up to 12 weeks
Mean change from baseline in total area of Choroidal Neovascularization (CNV) over 12 weeks		up to 12 weeks
The number of patients needing rescue treatment within 12 weeks		up to 12 weeks
The time to rescue treatment for needed patients within 12 weeks		up to 12 weeks
Incidence and severity of ocular and systemic adverse events		up to 12 weeks

Sponsor
Theratocular Biotek Co.

Collaborators
No information provided

Investigators
No information provided

General Publications
No publications available

Index

J. N. Weiss, *Clinical Trials in Age-Related Macular Degeneration Treatment*,
https://doi.org/10.1007/978-3-031-58803-7

GPSR Compliance

The European Union's (EU) General Product Safety Regulation (GPSR) is a set of rules that requires consumer products to be safe and our obligations to ensure this.

If you have any concerns about our products, you can contact us on ProductSafety@springernature.com

In case Publisher is established outside the EU, the EU authorized representative is:

Springer Nature Customer Service Center GmbH
Europaplatz 3
69115 Heidelberg, Germany

Batch number: 10726135

Printed by Printforce, the Netherlands